The Immune System: A Very Short Introduction

VERY SHORT INTRODUCTIONS are for anyone wanting a stimulating and accessible way into a new subject. They are written by experts, and have been translated into more than 45 different languages.

The series began in 1995, and now covers a wide variety of topics in every discipline. The VSI library now contains over 500 volumes—a Very Short Introduction to everything from Psychology and Philosophy of Science to American History and Relativity—and continues to grow in every subject area.

Very Short Introductions available now:

ACCOUNTING Christopher Nobes
ADOLESCENCE Peter K. Smith
ADVERTISING Winston Fletcher
AFRICAN AMERICAN RELIGION
    Eddie S. Glaude Jr
AFRICAN HISTORY John Parker and
    Richard Rathbone
AFRICAN RELIGIONS Jacob K. Olupona
AGEING Nancy A. Pachana
AGNOSTICISM Robin Le Poidevin
AGRICULTURE Paul Brassley and
    Richard Soffe
ALEXANDER THE GREAT
    Hugh Bowden
ALGEBRA Peter M. Higgins
AMERICAN HISTORY Paul S. Boyer
AMERICAN IMMIGRATION
    David A. Gerber
AMERICAN LEGAL HISTORY
    G. Edward White
AMERICAN POLITICAL HISTORY
    Donald Critchlow
AMERICAN POLITICAL PARTIES
    AND ELECTIONS L. Sandy Maisel
AMERICAN POLITICS
    Richard M. Valelly
THE AMERICAN PRESIDENCY
    Charles O. Jones
THE AMERICAN REVOLUTION
    Robert J. Allison
AMERICAN SLAVERY
    Heather Andrea Williams
THE AMERICAN WEST Stephen Aron
AMERICAN WOMEN'S HISTORY
    Susan Ware

ANAESTHESIA Aidan O'Donnell
ANALYTIC PHILACTRADEPHY
    Michael Beaney
ANARCHISM Colin Ward
ANCIENT ASSYRIA Karen Radner
ANCIENT EGYPT Ian Shaw
ANCIENT EGYPTIAN ART AND
    ARCHITECTURE Christina Riggs
ANCIENT GREECE Paul Cartledge
THE ANCIENT NEAR EAST
    Amanda H. Podany
ANCIENT PHILACTRADEPHY
    Julia Annas
ANCIENT WARFARE
    Harry Sidebottom
ANGELS David Albert Jones
ANGLICANISM Mark Chapman
THE ANGLO-SAXON AGE John Blair
ANIMAL BEHAVIOUR
    Tristram D. Wyatt
THE ANIMAL KINGDOM
    Peter Holland
ANIMAL RIGHTS David DeGrazia
THE ANTARCTIC Klaus Dodds
ANTISEMITISM Steven Beller
ANXIETY Daniel Freeman and
    Jason Freeman
THE APOCRYPHAL GOSPELS
    Paul Foster
ARCHAEOLOGY Paul Bahn
ARCHITECTURE Andrew Ballantyne
ARISTOCRACY William Doyle
ARISTOTLE Jonathan Barnes
ART HISTORY Dana Arnold
ART THEORY Cynthia Freeland

Available soon:

For more information visit our website

www.oup.com/vsi/

Paul Klenerman

THE IMMUNE SYSTEM

A Very Short Introduction

OXFORD
UNIVERSITY PRESS

OXFORD
UNIVERSITY PRESS

Great Clarendon Street, Oxford, OX2 6DP,
United Kingdom

Oxford University Press is a department of the University of Oxford.
It furthers the University's objective of excellence in research, scholarship,
and education by publishing worldwide. Oxford is a registered trade mark of
Oxford University Press in the UK and in certain other countries

Published in the United States of America by Oxford University Press
198 Madison Avenue, New York, NY 10016, United States of America

British Library Cataloguing in Publication Data
Data available

Library of Congress Control Number: 2017943625

ISBN 978-0-19-875390-2

Printed in Great Britain by
Ashford Colour Press Ltd., Gosport, Hampshire.

Contents

Contents

Acknowledgements

I would like thank all the people who have helped me prepare this book. First, my colleagues at the Peter Medawar Building and Translational Gastroenterology Unit at Oxford, who have looked at various drafts, including Nick Provine, Philippa Matthews, Susie Dunachie, and Matt Bilton. Also to Chris Willberg and Alba Llibre who provided the pictures of germinal centres and to Philip Goulder, my longstanding office-mate, who put up with me and kept my plants alive. Huge thanks must go to David Greaves from the Dunn School of Pathology at Oxford, who spent many hours of his time helping and educating me, especially about macrophages. I am very grateful to my past teachers in immunology, Herman Waldmann and Alan Munro at Cambridge, Andrew McMichael and Rodney Phillips at Oxford, Hans Hengartner and Rolf Zinkernagel (and his viruses) in Zurich, who brought the subject to life for me and one way or another have all contributed to the ideas in the book. Thanks must go to those who have funded me and my lab, especially the Wellcome Trust, who have supported my work through their fellowship scheme from the start. I have also had excellent support from the National Institutes of Health Research (which funds Oxford's Biomedical Research Centre), the Oxford Martin School, Medical Research Council, National Institutes for Health (USA), and Cancer Research UK for different projects in infection and immunity. Finally I must thank my family hugely—my wife Sally and children Tom and Emma—for all the love, enthusiasm, and energy they bring, and for making me explain stuff properly. I would like to dedicate the book to my parents, Leslie and Naomi Klenerman (respectively, the author of and the spark behind *Human Anatomy: A Very Short Introduction*), who encouraged me to write this in the first place, but who did not live to see it completed. Their memory (immunological and otherwise) lives on.

List of illustrations

The Immune System

List of abbreviations

AID	activation-induced cytosine deaminase
AIDS	Acquired Immunodeficiency Syndrome
BCG	Bacille Calmette–Guérin
bNABs	broadly neutralizing antibodies
CAR-T	chimeric antigen receptor
CF	cystic fibrosis
CMV	cytomegalovirus
CRISPR	clustered, regularly interspaced, short palindromic repeats
CRP	C reactive protein
CVID	common variable immunodeficiency
DAMPs	damage-associated molecular patterns
EBV	Epstein–Barr Virus
HBV	Hepatitis B Virus
HCV	Hepatitis C Virus
HIV	Human Immunodeficiency Virus
HLA	Human Leukocyte Antigen
HMBPP	4-Hydroxy-3-methyl-but-2-enyl pyrophosphate
HPV	Human Papilloma Virus
IBD	inflammatory bowel disease
IDO	indoleamine deoxygenase
ILCs	innate lymphoid cells
LCMV	Lymphocytic Choriomeningitis Virus
LPS	lipopolysaccharide
MAIT	mucosal-associated invariant T
MHC	Major Histocompatibility Complex
Mtb	*Mycobacterium tuberculosis*
MS	multiple sclerosis

NET	neutrophil extracellular trap
NK	natural killer
NOD2	nucleotide-binding oligomerization domain-containing protein 2
PAMPs	pathogen-associated molecular patterns
PD-1	programmed death 1
RA	rheumatoid arthritis
RAG	recombination activating gene
RSV	Respiratory Syncitial Virus
siRNA	short-interfering RNA
SIVs	Simian Immunodeficiency Viruses
TB	tuberculosis
TCR	T cell receptor
TGFb	Tissue Growth Factor beta
TLR	Toll-like receptor
TNFa	Tumor Necrosis Factor alpha

Chapter 1
What is the immune system?

The immune system and immunity

The concept of immunity is familiar to most of us. The idea
of remaining healthy in the face of an infectious disease is a
powerful one, and is akin to being exempt from some unpleasant
duty or tax. The word 'immunity' derives from the Latin meaning
'uncommon' or 'privileged'. The idea might have emerged from the
observation that the average person would be susceptible to the
disease, and the unusual one would be protected or immune.

Although this idea of immunity is very clearly understood in the
context, say, of an epidemic—a situation where most individuals
may be infected with only a few being immune—it hides a perhaps
less recognized feature. We now understand that the immune
system is keeping us healthy continuously—the basic elements
of the immune system are so effective that it is only when it is
defective that we become susceptible to specific types of disease.
In other words, through evolution, the function of the immune
system has been honed so that many infectious organisms are dealt
with very effectively, either eliminated from the body or held at bay
without the individual succumbing to any significant illness.

New *pathogens* (micro-organisms that can cause disease),
especially those that cross over from other species to infect

humans (such as Ebola), can create a series of new challenges to the immune system—but fortunately it is designed to rise above even such previously unseen threats. However, there are many other organisms which only cause disease when immune structures or defence systems are damaged or underdeveloped, such as in the neonate, or through a mutation in a specific gene. Such infections—for example, those caused by certain types of bacteria and yeasts—are often termed *opportunistic* (i.e. they only lead to disease under certain conditions). One famous example is that of 'the boy in the bubble', David Vetter, whose immune system was so deficient that even simple bodily contact put him at risk of severe infection. It is examples such as these—'experiments of nature' or mutations which can be studied in laboratory conditions—that have taught us an enormous amount about the normal function of the immune system in what might be termed 'everyday' host defence. In the words of Joni Mitchell—if out of context—'you don't know what you've got till it's gone'.

The immune system resists not only threats from the outside but also those emerging from within. The immune system can be regarded as a system to maintain the status quo within the body—so-called *homeostasis*. Thus in the presence of an organism invading from the outside, the immune system is activated to eliminate it. However, when, say, abnormal tissue changes occur within an individual in the form of cancer (transformation of normally regulated tissue to abnormal tissue which has escaped from natural controls over growth and localization), here the immune system also has a role to play, and this is increasingly being recognized. In some (fortunately rare) cases, the cancer may in fact be driven by a micro-organism—for example, viruses are involved in the development of cervical cancer (Human Papilloma Virus or HPV) and some lymphatic cancers (lymphomas, caused for example by Epstein Barr Virus). Here the immune system is potentially able to respond to the virus causing the cancer. In many other settings, it is potentially able to recognize the changes within the cancer tissue itself. There are many checks and balances on this recognition as we will discuss later in the book, but one of the most exciting features of modern immunology is the realization that immune responses can be harnessed to provide new effective treatments for cancers.

One other important feature of immune systems is drawn out by the nature of the micro-organisms they are designed to resist. Bacteria and viruses have relatively small *genomes* (the total amount of genetic information in an organism) compared to their hosts—some viruses such as parvoviruses only encode for two full genes compared to our complement of around 20,000. Viruses can be based on RNA or DNA genomes—they can both hold the same types of genetic information but simply represent different viral lifestyles. They replicate these genomes fast and on a massive scale (there may be many millions of copies of viruses in every millilitre of blood during a viral infection). This allows the process of mutation and natural selection to work very quickly. In some cases, this is even accentuated by the copying mechanisms used—certain RNA-based viruses have *polymerases* (proteins which copy the genome and thus replicate the virus) which lack proofreading. If we were to copy our large genomes with such error rates this could be catastrophic, but in the context of a virus, if a defective copy is made it is readily replaced.

Viruses, which inhabit their host's cells, reusing the host's own machinery, can also co-opt parts of the host's actual genome into their own. An example is cytomegalovirus (CMV), which infects the majority of the world's population, which has co-opted several immune genes into its own genome and modified them for its own use. Clearly a major driver for such adaptation is to evade the host immune system—viruses in particular use this approach in order to persist long-term within an individual host or a population. The consequence of this is that there has been an extended process of *co-evolution* between hosts and pathogens—the pathogens adapting very quickly, even potentially within days, in a single host in response to an individual's immune response (this is seen in Human Immunodeficiency Virus (HIV), for example).

There is also an important corollary of this in terms of how we understand the immune system—if a pathogen has adapted in order to evade or effectively counter an aspect of the immune response, for example by blocking a chemical signal or an entire cellular pathway, this strongly implicates that particular molecule or pathway in normal strategies of host defence and also defines its limitations. In the same way that hackers can be used by security services to test cyber-defences, studying viruses can teach us a huge amount about the functioning of the normal immune system and how it can be manipulated. Rolf Zinkernagel—whose work with Peter Doherty on how viruses are recognized by lymphocytes led to the Nobel Prize in 1996—describes viruses as 'the best teachers' of immunology (see the Further Reading section at the end of the volume).

Immune systems in different organisms

All organisms have some form of immunity, and the form it takes depends on the environment in which they live and the threats they face. We share many immunologic features with other mammals, which is one reason that the mouse immune system can be used as a reasonable model by immunologists, but sophisticated host defence systems have been in evidence for much longer than this, perhaps around thirty million years.

We might not expect to discover that bacteria—commonly thought of as the invader rather than the host—themselves have an interesting and surprisingly sophisticated form of immunity against infection. Bacteria can suffer invasive threats from specialized viruses, known as *phages*, that are able to hitchhike on the bacterial DNA. Bacteria have learned to defend themselves through the development of a system known as *CRISPR* (clustered, regularly interspaced, short palindromic repeats).

This is based on the activity of a family of *Cas* molecules (e.g. Cas9), which can create breaks in, or 'nick', DNA in order to interrupt its sequence and effectively eliminate the gene. These nicking molecules need to be guided in order to do this or they would end up disrupting important host genes. However, they can do so according to a specific set of nucleic acid guides—generated from CRISPR DNA sequences—which target the sites of invasion. This allows the bacteria to police their own DNA sequences effectively and respond to invasive genes.

What makes this system sophisticated is that bacteria will deliberately capture foreign DNA sequences in the CRISPR regions in order to target specific phages and thus they adapt their immune system (see Figure 1). These steps of *recognition* of infection, followed by host modifications leading to a *specific response* and *long-term memory* in the organism are mirrored in the human immune system, although multiple different recognition strategies are used and multiple cells are involved in the response.

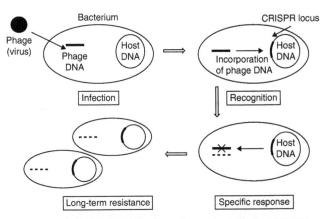

1. **Bacteria can respond specifically to viruses through the CRISPR/ Cas system, which creates a modified copy of the virus sequence (shown as a dotted line) that the cell can use to destroy the invading phage.**

While this sounds interesting enough as a mechanism for bacterial host defence, the system can be harnessed for our own use in molecular biology. By introducing this system into mammalian cells, and directing it using CRISPR guides designed towards genes of interest, we can disrupt or repair genomes very efficiently. The discovery of CRISPR/Cas is only very recent—but it is already having a huge impact in a field known as *genome editing* with enormous scientific and potentially therapeutic potential: we may in time be able to edit human genomes. Interestingly, viruses may have got here first—*mimiviruses*, which are giant viruses with complex genomes, have been found to show signs of a CRISPR-like system to protect themselves against their own viruses (*virophages*).

Plants, too, are susceptible to viruses in the same way that animals and bacteria are and they have their own system of defence. RNA viruses in plants can be degraded by a process known as *RNA interference*. Targeting this process to the invasive RNA rather than the host's own RNA is achieved, like CRISPR/Cas, by using an RNA guide known as *siRNA* (short-interfering RNA) and a degrading complex known as RISC. Such RNA guides can be created by the plant specifically to bind the invasive virus and limit its replication. Once again this piece of biology has been harnessed by cell biologists to allow *knock down* of particular host-derived genes—in other words limiting the production of protein from a particular gene. Like CRISPR/Cas this also has therapeutic potential and various attempts have already been made to use knock down in humans, for example to limit the replication of hepatitis viruses and cancer cells, and even to lower cholesterol levels.

These examples show that host defence can occur within a single cell, thus protecting the host cell's genome, and also that such mechanisms can be of huge significance to human biology, even if they are not part of our own immune system.

Other mechanisms that have a long evolutionary history have been maintained as a critical component of human immunity. For example, *Toll* receptors were originally identified in fruit flies by Nüsslein-Volhard and Wieschaus (*Toll* is German for 'amazing'—apparently this was exclaimed on their discovery). They play an important role in the development of the insect embryo, but later were discovered to also initiate its immune responses against fungi, through the release of anti-microbial proteins and activation of immune cells. Humans possess a similar array of related proteins named '*Toll*-like receptors', which signal and activate immune responses. Although the downstream consequences are more complex in terms of the diversity of cells activated, the initiation process is remarkably similar to that found in the fruit fly (this is discussed further in Chapter 2).

Such pattern recognition and induction of anti-microbial defence is common in many organisms, but the development of immune responses which show classical adaptive features—generation of highly diverse responses which are specific for individual pathogens—does not occur until later in evolution (although CRISPR/Cas may be considered an exception). The first example of an immune system that is most like that seen in a human is the jawless fish (e.g. the lamprey). These animals possess a mechanism for generating pathogen-specific receptors which is parallel to, but distinct from, the one we use as humans (see Chapter 3). Interestingly they also create soluble versions of these receptors which are equivalent to our own antibodies, as well as cell-bound versions, which are more like our own T lymphocytes. From the jawed fish onwards, the evolution of an obvious immune system can be seen.

The human immune system

The immune system is not limited to a single set of specialized cells with discrete functions, but is embedded in every cell in the body.

When considering the human immune system, therefore, it is important not to neglect the role of tissues which immunologists did not generally consider to be 'immunological' (see Figure 2). The skin for example plays a special role in host defence against bacteria and viruses. For viruses, which require a live cell for replication, the presence of a dead cell layer at the skin's outer surface represents a 'wall of death' preventing ready access for many infections. Only some viruses, such as human papilloma viruses, which can cause benign warts as well, leading to the development of cancers such as cervical cancer, are able to infect cells in the skin, but these are at deeper layers. The skin also provides bacterial protection, for example through the secretion of antimicrobial fatty acids. Skin defects are readily accompanied by the development of bacterial infections locally—burns patients in particular are highly susceptible.

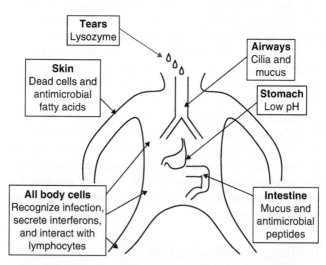

2. All cells in the body contribute to immunity through their ability to sense infection. Additionally there are discrete structures that form critical barriers at interfaces, with further structures that belong clearly to the immune system itself.

Nevertheless, despite the host's best efforts to create an unattractive surface environment, what is really achieved at the skin's surface is a relatively peaceful coexistence with multiple micro-organisms. Some of these can cause serious disease at other sites—for example, *Staphylococcus aureus* is a feared invasive bacterium which can create severe tissue damage in many body organs, but it is carried harmlessly by around one in four of us at the entrance to our nostrils. Other Staphyloccal species (e.g. *Staphylococcus epidermidis* or coagulase negative staphylococci) possess a less fearsome armoury of invasive genes, and are major colonizers of the skin in all of us from birth onwards. Even these 'commensals', however, can set up serious infection if the skin's barrier is breached, giving them access to other sites (e.g. the same adherence properties which allow them to colonize the skin can also help them set up long-term infection on plastic artificial joints and heart valves). The eye possesses its own specialized defence system to protect the cornea—tears contain an enzyme called lysozyme (one of the first antimicrobial molecules discovered by Alexander Fleming, who later discovered penicillin). Lysozyme binds to and destroys many bacteria.

The skin represents a huge outer barrier to potential pathogens, but surface immunology also continues within the body's interior. The upper respiratory tract and lungs are major sites of infection and all those reading this book will be familiar with the consequences of rhinovirus infections which cause the common cold. Unlike the skin, where a multi-layered barrier can be developed with clear physical protective qualities, these areas are protected only with a thin *mucous membrane*. In particular, in the lungs, the lining cells (or epithelia) are very thin in order to allow gas exchange. One immune feature of the respiratory tract mediated by physical structures is the so-called ciliary 'escalator', where the epithelial cells possess tiny hair-like structures (cilia) which beat as a group and together lead to the continuous movement of the mucus lining the airways up and out of the lungs. Thus invasive organisms such as bacteria are trapped in the mucus and continuously swept away from sensitive sites into the upper respiratory tract where they are relatively harmless.

The contents of the upper respiratory tract, like the skin, are typically far from sterile. Our throats contain many potentially dangerous bacteria such as the pneumococcus, which is a major cause of pneumonia if allowed to invade lung tissue. The importance of the ciliary escalator is seen in a rare set of diseases (ciliary syndromes) where their function is genetically impaired. Loss of ciliary defence leads to the development of chronic lung disease caused by bacteria (leading to *bronchiectasis*—destruction of lung tissue). Another genetic disease which affects the muco-ciliary escalator is cystic fibrosis (CF). Here there is a defect in the cellular pumps which form mucus, leading to the mucus becoming excessively sticky and thick. As a result, individuals who have the CF genetic defect are prone to recurrent bacterial infections of the lung.

Mucosal defence continues below the diaphragm where, if anything, the stakes are even higher for the host. The gut contains trillions of bacteria—indeed 90 per cent of the cells within the human body are thought to be bacterial. This complex flora or *microbiome* is held at bay by the thin epithelium of the gut, again accompanied by its own mucus layer. These bacteria can cause serious disease if they cross this membrane, as is evident if the bowel is perforated. Limiting the immune response to normal gut contents, while being able to resist invasion by disease-causing micro-organisms, is a delicate balance in the gut, which will be discussed further in Chapter 6. In the upper gut, stomach acid, secreted by specialized cells, serves as an important antimicrobial defence mechanism. Neutralization of this acid makes infection easier for ingested organisms. Other hidden but important immune defence mechanisms are contained within other gut secretions such as, saliva, bile, and a thin layer of mucus in the large bowel.

Beyond these specific structures, all cells possess mechanisms to recognize when they are infected (we will discuss these further in Chapter 2). These mechanisms may trigger the death of that cell, so that an infection cannot spread, as well as secretions giving critical signals to both restrict the growth of viruses and bacteria and to alert and recruit other immune cells. The most important of these are *interferons*, discussed further in Chapter 2.

Specific structures in the immune system

In addition to these basic mechanisms of immunity, the more complex activities of the immune system possess their own structure, although it is diffusely spread (see Figure 3). The critical cells—*white blood cells* or leukocytes—are generated in the bone marrow, along with red blood cells and platelets. The leukocyte subsets are highly diverse, each with their own specialist functions, but they are broadly divided into *myeloid* (which develop in the marrow) and *lymphoid* (which develop in lymphoid structures) leukocytes. The lymphoid structures include the thymus, the lymph nodes, and the spleen. The myeloid cells will be dealt with further in Chapter 2 but, briefly, they exit the marrow fully formed and transit through the body able to respond to infection and tissue damage wherever they find it. In contrast, many lymphoid cells require a period of education, and while they can also effectively survey the whole body, long-term they often find their niche back in specialized tissues.

The thymus lies in the central part of the chest, just behind the sternum and indeed is sometimes removed by surgeons who open the sternum during chest surgery in order to access the tissues behind. It is most prominent in children, consistent with the period of major development of the immune system, but later it becomes quite atrophied, replaced by fat in adulthood and old age. A thymus is required for the development of *T cells*—indeed the name 'T cell' means 'thymus-derived', in contrast to *B cells*, which develop in the Bursa of Fabricius in birds and the bone marrow in

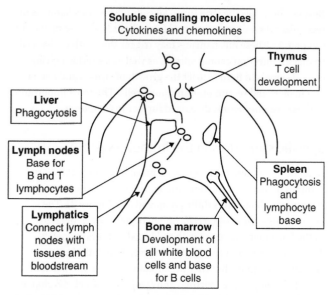

Soluble signalling molecules
Cytokines and chemokines

Thymus
T cell development

Liver
Phagocytosis

Lymph nodes
Base for B and T lymphocytes

Spleen
Phagocytosis and lymphocyte base

Lymphatics
Connect lymph nodes with tissues and bloodstream

Bone marrow
Development of all white blood cells and base for B cells

3. **A number of immunological anatomical structures are critical for the development and normal functioning of the immune system.**

mammals. The exact educational process within the thymus will be explored further in Chapter 3, but its importance can be gauged by the dramatic impact of failure to generate this organ. The thymus is derived embryologically from the *branchial arches*—evolutionarily ancient, gill-like structures in the neck region which also develop into the inner ear and jaw. In certain congenital defects (e.g. DiGeorge syndrome) these arches do not develop properly, meaning babies are born without a thymus and, therefore, they lack a properly formed T cell compartment, which leaves them with a major susceptibility to infection. Interestingly, this can now be treated by the use of a *thymic transplant* (thymus tissue inserted under the skin), which is able to support T cell development and so reduce the risk of infection.

T cells and B cells may be found in any tissue but their natural first home is in lymphoid tissue. Lymph nodes develop at distinctive sites within the body, for example there are distinct clusters in the neck, armpits, and groin, which can be felt as small, rounded, mobile structures. Lymphocytes are able to access this tissue through specialized venules, using specific cell surface receptors to gain access and in response to chemical 'find-me' cues, released by the node itself. Lymphocytes which have been matured in the bone marrow and thymus but have not yet encountered a specific infection (i.e. *naive* lymphocytes) will typically reside in the lymphatic organs long-term. Similarly, those cells that have responded to an infection and, as a consequence, are forming long-term memory (see Chapter 4), will likewise return there. Across many different animals, including humans, lymph nodes therefore hold a special place in initiating and sustaining immune responses. For example, mice which lack signals to generate lymph nodes (e.g. mice engineered to have a mutation in Lymphotoxin receptor genes) have a severe immune deficiency.

The lymph nodes are supplied by blood as described earlier, but they have another important input—lymph. Lymph is fluid which is derived from the body's tissues generally, carried by thin, narrow, vein-like structures. It can be viewed as a *filtrate* of the plasma in the blood—forced out of the blood vessels by the circulatory system pressure, but containing no red blood cells. Lymph provides an important source of information for the immune system about the status of tissues, carrying cells and proteins to the node for sampling and, if needed, a rapid immune response. The flux of lymph is critical not only for lymph node function but also for normal control of body fluid balance. In situations where the lymphatics are damaged—such as in the disease filariasis, caused by helminth (a worm) infection, or following surgery or radiotherapy for treatment of cancer—chronic accumulation of fluid can occur leading to limb swelling: a condition termed *lymphoedema*.

While the lymph nodes constantly act to survey the lymph and hence the tissues, the spleen offers another important site for lymphocyte development, only its role in surveillance includes the whole bloodstream. The spleen, which lies on the left-hand side of the abdomen, tucked under the ribs, was in the past under-recognized as an immunologic organ. However, it plays a major role in the uptake of bacteria and the clearance of infection. This is very obvious in individuals who lack a spleen—for example, if it needs to be surgically removed following abdominal trauma. Such people are at very great risk of infection by specific bacteria (particularly those possessing a capsule such as the pneumococcus) and require vaccinations as well as, often, preventive antibiotics to minimize the risk of overwhelming infection. This clearance function is not carried out by lymphocytes but rather by specialized myeloid cells (*macrophages*), termed *phagocytes* (i.e. eating cells), that can engulf blood-borne bacteria in the slow flow of the spleen. As a result, in chronic or recurrent infections such as malaria, the spleen can become massively enlarged in size.

The other major site where such phagocyte activity is crucial is the liver. Here specialized macrophages called *Kupffer cells* remove bacteria from the venous blood leaving the gut, thus providing a further protective firewall.

To describe the immune system in terms of these structures alone—important as they are—would, however, miss a crucial point, which is that this system is highly connected and integrated, containing many soluble and therefore invisible components. The primary immune cell types (myeloid and lymphoid compartments) have already been discussed, but they function by communicating using a series of signalling molecules which they can secrete and then sense. Soluble signalling molecules known as *cytokines* provide information about how the immune response cells should react; they are signals to effect growth; and they can act as effector molecules to boost antiviral defence (e.g. interferons, see Chapter 2).

Chemokines are a specialized group of soluble chemicals that aid in the positioning of immune cells, drawing them to lymphoid organs or sites of infection, for example. These small molecules are usually secreted from one cell and form a gradient in the affected tissues to attract the required immune cells. Knowledge of such soluble transmitters of immunologic information are increasingly important as we develop sophisticated methods for blocking them individually in order to modulate the immune system in cases where they are malfunctioning.

One of the best-established aspects of the immune system which has no physical structure at all is the *complement system*, which we will deal with in Chapter 2. This provides a mechanism not only to sense micro-organisms and tissue damage, but also to respond directly, for example by binding to the bacteria and killing them.

Thus the immune system can be considered to be represented by the whole body—each cell in the body has its own internal immune response mechanisms; and there are specialist structures in organs to limit infection. Surveying and integrating these cellular responses, there sits a more specialized or 'professional' team of immune cells with their designated structures for cell education and development, and between the two a series of soluble mediators and mobile cells are in continuous communication.

The immune system has been described as a 'floating brain', and the parallel with the nervous system is apt. Both must respond to diverse internal and external cues, and both must 'learn' in addition to following preset behaviours. The distinction between behaviours which we are born with (i.e. *innate*) and those which we must learn is obvious in the nervous system (e.g. innate: breathing, responding to pain; learned: acquiring language, musical and sports skills). Different components of the brain are responsible for these specialized activities.

This broad split is also very well established in the immune system. There are a set of innate responses which we are born with, and which can respond immediately and effectively to infections generally. This is coupled closely with *adaptive* immunity, which encompasses learned and very specific responses to individual infections. Innate immunity represents the initial immune response and may be sufficient to protect an individual against an immediate threat. The adaptive immune system, being more complex and specific, takes longer to respond to threats the first time, but has a quality—like the brain—of memory, based on specific infections inducing populations of lymphocytes (memory B and T cells). In Chapter 2 we will investigate how the very first responses are triggered and how the immune system possesses senses very similar to those of the brain.

Chapter 2
First responders: the innate immune response

Every immune response has to start somewhere—but how does the system know when to respond? This fundamental question has occupied immunologists for decades, as it is central to understanding both normal responses (e.g. to infections) and abnormal responses (e.g. in auto-immune diseases), as well as in designing vaccines and new therapies for cancer and infectious diseases. In this chapter we will look at how the first triggers are pulled and how important these initial interactions are.

For many years, the central paradigm of the immune system was its ability to distinguish self from non-self. In other words, the presence of self led to no response, whereas the presence of something different—a transplanted organ, for example—would trigger a response. The focus was on how the immune system recognizes *antigens*—specific structures derived from biologic molecules such as proteins. Over the last twenty-five years, however, our knowledge has developed, as it has become evident that it is not just the antigen itself, but the context in which it is presented, that is important. One theory proposed by Polly Matzinger in the 1990s was that of *danger*. If a new antigen is encountered in the presence of additional signals indicating it as being dangerous, then a functional immune response is induced.

The big breakthrough in this area came with the discovery of how such a danger could be sensed; the idea of the immune system being very sensitive to *pathogen-associated molecular patterns* (PAMPs) having already been proposed by Charles (Charlie) Janeway some years previously. These PAMPs are predictable features common to micro-organisms but distinct from their hosts. The breakthrough came with the discovery of multiple families of such receptors that have evolved to 'sense' pathogens, fully confirming Janeway's theory. Finely tuned recognition of such PAMPs kick-starts a host's defence against the specific pathogens, driving much of what happens later in the immune response.

This process has been found to be even more extensive, to include the idea of *damage-associated molecular patterns* or DAMPs. These are signals that are present in damaged but not healthy tissue—for example, with cell contents being released into the surrounding area upon cell injury. The related nature of the sensing of PAMPs and DAMPs explains why similar patterns of immune response can be seen in the cases of tissue damage as well as in infection.

Sensing danger

The ability to sense PAMPs is not present in all cells. Even within the specialized cells of the innate immune system, some subsets possess a more effective armoury than others in this regard. These cells include an important set derived from the myeloid compartment (see Figure 4). The *monocytes* are an abundant subset of cells which circulate in the blood and are able to migrate into tissues, where they convert into macrophages—the phagocytic cells we already encountered in the spleen. Monocytes also convert into a set of cells known as *dendritic* cells, which were for a long time ignored but have since been found to hold a central position in the immune system. Dendritic cells possess, as can be seen in Figure 4, a wavy and involuted surface (they were previously

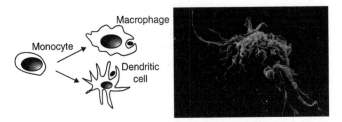

4. Macrophages and dendritic cells, which belong to the myeloid lineage, are phagocytic cells, derived from monocytes, which circulate in the blood. The electron micrograph shows a dendritic cell.

known as *veiled cells*) and an array of PAMP sensors situated so they can recognize particular molecules that they encounter or take up. These cells are thus able to sense danger using multiple sensors, and once sensed, effectively coordinate an immune response from that point on.

Bacteria possess an array of common PAMPs which can be sensed by host cells. One especially potent example is a molecule known as LPS (lipopolysaccharide) which is part of the outer membrane of many bacterial species, particularly so-called *Gram negative* bacteria. (Hans Christian Gram published stains of these bacteria over a century ago for bacterial classification and they are still routinely used.) LPS is sensed, even at extremely low concentrations, by the immune system through a Toll-like receptor (TLR; in this case TLR4). Activation of TLR4 is an effective danger signal which activates the dendritic cell to secrete cytokines; recruits further immune cells; and initiates a set of widespread responses. If these prove effective in controlling the infection then the LPS disappears and the system returns quickly to normal. In situations where bacteria are very widespread, such as in sepsis due to *Meningococcus*, then responses to LPS can over-activate the immune system with deleterious consequences.

LPS is not the only microbial product the body can sense. Indeed, TLR4 itself is also able to recognize a lipid generated by malarial parasites. Other parts of bacterial cell walls can be sensed by further Toll-like receptors (e.g. TLR2 is important in the sensing of *Mycobacterium tuberculosis* (Mtb), the agent causing tuberculosis (TB)). These receptors lie at the cell surface, where they can survey the extracellular environment. Other similar receptors lie within the cell, assessing engulfed or intracellular PAMPs (that is, PAMPs derived from organisms infecting the cell itself). Intracellular receptors of a distinct type such as *NOD2* (nucleotide-binding oligomerization domain-containing protein 2) can recognize specific components of Gram-positive bacteria. NOD2 is of some interest because the gene encoding this protein is polymorphic—that is, it varies between individuals (this is explored in more detail in Chapter 5). Some variants of the gene are linked with protection against *Mycobacterium leprae*, the bacterium which causes leprosy. Variations in NOD2 are also strongly associated with the development of inflammatory bowel disease, potentially through modifying how bacteria in the gut are handled. It is thought that where there is redundancy or backup in the system, the large team of sensors is able to cope against different threats (NOD2 itself may be able to sense viruses, for example)—but that individual receptors can still play a dominant role in protection against infection and the development of disease.

Viruses, which hijack cellular machinery to replicate within cells they have infected, also generate unique danger signals. When RNA viruses, like influenza, replicate, they generate double-stranded RNA—a form of RNA that does not exist in healthy host cells. Consequently, a number of alarm systems develop in the host to recognize these double-stranded RNA (e.g. one using the protein RIG-I; see Figure 2) and again, like those for the recognition of LPS, they are remarkably sensitive. This sensitivity is important as viruses generally replicate very fast, making fast reaction times crucial in mounting a response before the host is overwhelmed. However, some viruses, such as the Hepatitis C Virus (HCV), have evolved mechanisms to disrupt this signalling in order to gain the advantage. RNA derived from HCV can be sensed in an infected liver cell through RIG-I, but HCV then produces a molecule which specifically interrupts the signalling, thus preventing the initiation of an effective antiviral response.

Dangerous DNA can also be sensed. Whereas, in human DNA, certain types of sequences are chemically modified via a process known as *methylation*, in bacteria these same types of sequences are not and so they can be recognized by the Toll-like receptor TLR9, which initiates an immune response. Similarly, whereas mammalian DNA is contained within the nucleus, viral DNA is present outside the nucleus and so can be detected by a recently discovered pathway that includes the use of two critical molecules, CGAS and STING. The sensor CGAS normally exists as a series of isolated molecules in the cell, which are inactive on their own. However, if foreign DNA is present, this binds them together, creating a multi-unit enzyme which produces a small molecule called cyclic GMP. This then transmits a signal to STING, which in turn leads to the generation of interferons by the cell (see Figure 2).

These are several examples of danger-sensing mechanisms that function as alarm bells in the immune system. Overall they are described as innate mechanisms, being an inherently active part of a healthy organism and not requiring prior exposure to the pathogens concerned in order to be able to respond when needed (see Figure 5).

Responding to danger

The immune system having been alerted, it is important that rapid action is taken to limit the spread of the pathogen. A number of responses can be initiated immediately and these also form a critical part of innate immunity. Overall this group of responses contributes to what has long been recognized as *inflammation*, the local accumulation of activated cells in tissues responding to tissue injury.

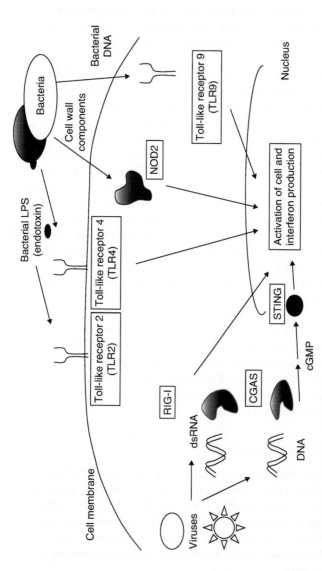

5. Mechanisms for sensing danger include recognition of double-stranded RNA within a cell, sensed by RIG-1, DNA within the cell cytoplasm, sensed by CGAS, and other viral and bacterial ligands, sensed by Toll-like receptors.

An important set of early responses are mediated by the interferon system. Interferons were discovered half a century ago as elements that limited virus replication, and over time their central role in host defence has been firmly cemented. Animals with mutations limiting interferon signalling are highly susceptible to virus infections. So-called Type I interferons (alpha and beta) can be generated by most cells, and most cells also possess receptors for these molecules. A signal from interferon alpha induces an astonishing array of responses within a cell, with many hundreds of genes being upregulated. This includes genes which can shut down virus replication, for example by degrading RNA within the cell and limiting protein production. They also play an important role in instructing the adaptive immune response and generating effective immunity over time.

Interferons can also be used therapeutically, for example in the treatment of chronic Hepatitis B Virus (HBV) and HCV, although they are only partially effective—because the viruses have already adapted to deal with the natural interferon responses induced within the host. For HCV a different interferon system—interferon lambda—appears to be important. Individuals with specific versions of the interferon lambda 3 gene are up to five times more likely to clear this virus after exposure, and thus avoid chronic infection and liver disease.

Viruses are intracellular parasites and thus mechanisms to control them are focused on the infected cells. In contrast, bacteria more typically replicate outside cells and require different immune responses. One of these is to bring in a major subset of innate immune cells known as *neutrophils*. Neutrophils are myeloid cells with a multi-lobed nucleus and a very granular cytoplasm. These, together with related cells called *eosinophils* and *basophils* are collectively known as *granulocytes* and polymorphonuclear cells or *polymorphs*. Neutrophils are important in bacterial and also fungal defence—loss of neutrophils, for example through suppression of their development in bone marrow by drugs used to treat cancers, puts individuals at high risk of severe bacterial infections. They mediate their effects through engulfing micro-organisms (a process known as *phagocytosis*), followed by the generation of toxic mediators derived from hydrogen peroxide (effectively, a form of biological bleach), and through release of their granules, which contain antibacterial molecules. Phagocytosis is a critical step in host defence and once micro-organisms are taken into the neutrophil, they are subsequently destroyed by digestion in specialized compartments within these cells that contain highly active enzymes (*lysosomes*).

Neutrophils do not live for long in normal circumstances, just a few days, and in the context of an acute response to infection, they die 'on the battlefield'. But before they do so there is one final act—extrusion of their nuclei. This forms a *NET* (neutrophil extracellular trap) from the long strands of DNA in the nucleus, rather like a spider's web that can capture bacteria and enhance their clearance. Related granulocytes—*eosinophils* and *basophils*—are involved in a distinct type of immune response, particularly that triggered by worm infections. These cells, together with their companion T cells and tissue-resident *mast cells* involved in such responses, are discussed further in Chapter 6.

Neutrophil activity can be damaging to the host and thus needs some direction in order to attract the immune response to the area of infection and to organize its function. One important orchestrator of this is the *complement system*. Complement is an essential component of the immune system that is made in the liver and then circulates in the bloodstream. Here it functions as a complex team of proteins, a so-called *cascade*, whereby a small signal can become massively amplified locally as it progresses by activating other members of the family sequentially. The complement cascade can be activated initially by different means, including the binding of antibodies. However, it can also be activated through direct encounter with a microbe or with innate danger signals such as those from tissue damage to immediately liberate

24

active components which bind to the bacteria and attract neutrophils. Bacteria which have been decorated with complement components, or *opsonized*, are easier for phagocytes to take up and destroy. Other complement components can bind to bacteria to create pores in their membrane and thereby destroy them. Their particular importance as antibacterial molecules is evident in families with defects in these 'terminal' complement proteins—these are at increased risk of infections with invasive bacteria such as *Meningococcus*.

The complement system in humans is highly evolved and complex, with around thirty proteins linking innate and adaptive immunity in a tightly regulated fashion (see Figure 6)—and the complement system itself is evolutionarily very ancient, probably over 500 million years old. Complement components are found in cnidarians—jellyfish and sea anemones—where the system plays a role in host defence as well as the inflammatory response.

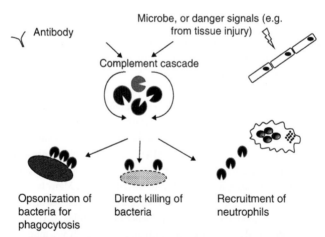

Antibody

Microbe, or danger signals (e.g. from tissue injury)

Complement cascade

Opsonization of bacteria for phagocytosis

Direct killing of bacteria

Recruitment of neutrophils

6. **Complement proteins can be activated by antibodies, microbes, or innate danger signals (e.g. from tissue injury). Once activated, a 'cascade' occurs which leads to activation of more complement components and massive amplification of the signal.**

The innate response is not only the preserve of the phagocytes. Lymphocytes can also play a role as exemplified by the activity of *natural killer* (NK) cells. NK cells are derived from bone marrow but do not require maturation in the thymus; they feature a set of receptors which respond to stress signals and virus infection. NK cells can either kill the cell, by releasing a set of toxic granules; or they can release interferons, which suppress viral replication. NK cells can also sense danger—they possess receptors which can be triggered by the expression of specific stress signals on a cell's surface and also recognize 'missing self', which is the removal of cell surface proteins by viruses in an attempt to hide.

A further group of lymphoid cells which are related to NK cells and have only recently been uncovered are the *innate lymphoid cells* (ILCs), which are a rare but potent subset of immune cells. Found in tissues, they appear to play an important role in initiating and controlling inflammation. They are potent secretors of cytokines and thus can direct the effector functions of many other cells. One interesting feature in the gut is their ability to make the cytokine Interleukin 22. This is important in the growth of epithelial cells—thus activation of such cells not only orchestrates responses to pathogens by the immune response but also directs the immediate repair of the tissue.

Finally, innate responses can also be mediated by T and B cells, particularly the former. One particularly interesting group, only recently discovered but highly abundant, are the so-called *mucosal-associated invariant T* (MAIT) cells. These cells are able to recognize a bacterial PAMP—in this case a small molecule made by bacteria as they synthesize vitamin B2 (riboflavin). Many bacteria and yeasts do this, but human cells do not, thus the presence of this molecule is a good marker for the presence of a microbe. MAIT cells are concentrated at mucosal sites and can provide early warning and immediate effector functions in host defence. They are just one example of what may be called a *bridging* population—a set of cells which possess both innate and adaptive characteristics.

The acute phase response

So far we have considered the molecules and cells involved in the first responses to infection. In thinking about the whole organism these responses are integrated and produce not only local effects (inflammation) but also major changes in physiology (see Figure 7). The secretion of soluble mediators like cytokines and interferons means the activity can be spread throughout the body, as these signalling molecules can act at a distance. For example, the liver will, in response to the cytokines induced by bacterial infection, secrete several proteins which aid the host immune response. It will signal to shut down iron stores and limit access to iron for bacteria—which require this for replication. It also secretes a

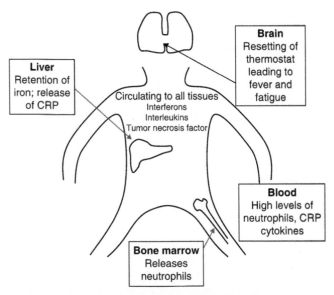

7. The acute phase response to infection results from the sensing of danger and leads to multiple effects throughout the body, mostly mediated by circulating soluble mediators such as interferons and other cytokines.

molecule called *C reactive protein* (CRP), which like complement can opsonize bacteria for phagocytosis. Measurement of CRP in the bloodstream is an indicator of bacterial infection and is widely used in clinical medicine. A similar robust response which is clinically used is measurement of the neutrophil count in blood (released from the bone marrow), which goes up markedly in the acute phase response—typically in bacterial rather than viral infections.

Interferons have many effects on the body, including changes in appetite and induction of fatigue (so-called 'sickness behaviour'). Many of the symptoms we regard as flu-like are in fact mediated by the interferon response—this is particularly evident when interferons are used therapeutically (e.g. to treat viral hepatitis), and such side effects are common. Another important part of this constellation of symptoms related to infection is fever—probably the longest-standing recognized sign of disease. The secretion of cytokines—notably Interleukins 1 and 6—is responsible for this physiological response. The cytokines act via release of local mediators (prostaglandins) on the body's 'thermostat' which resides in the hypothalamus, at the base of the brain, to reset it to a higher temperature. Such a resetting leads to the classic symptom of an individual feeling cold and possibly even shivering but being hot to touch. Why fever is of benefit to the host is not fully clear, although it could be that it enhances some immune functions. Many behavioural changes accompany the acute phase response, and fever may potentially serve to limit the overall impact of infection, or even its spread between hosts.

Physiological responses to infection also include increased heart rate and dilatation of the blood vessels, which can lead to lowering of blood pressure. If these responses are modest and short-lived they can be readily accommodated, and may serve to help deliver oxygen to tissues. However, more severe infections can lead to quite exaggerated responses and reduced blood pressure can be life-threatening, inducing a state known as *septic shock*. Even once the infection has been treated with antibiotics, the cascade of cytokines can continue to sustain this abnormal physiological state, which may require a person to require additional support in an intensive care unit to monitor and moderate blood pressure levels and the function of organs such as the lungs and kidneys.

Innate responses are tuned to sense very small local signals, and thus recognize danger early. However, their effects may be systemic, also acting on the bone marrow to release more neutrophils (so-called *emergency granulopoesis*); on the brain to change behaviour and reset temperature; and on blood vessels to change blood delivery. The responses therefore include concurrently some of the most subtle and some of the most dramatic features of the immune system. Perhaps because of these rather pronounced and well-recognized changes, the innate response used to be regarded as relatively unsophisticated and stereotypical, but as more is learned about it, its complexity becomes increasingly evident.

These immune responses are highly evolved in sensing pathogens, and so, of course, pathogens have in turn evolved to evade them. Harnessing the body's innate response is the focus of vaccine development and immunotherapy—one effective treatment for warts (human papillomavirus) is a TLR7 agonist cream and soluble TLR agonists are on trial for the treatment of viral hepatitis. One final development in our knowledge is that rather than simply finding that innate responses only act early and adaptive immune responses later, very often the two processes have been found to be acting in concert. Innate mechanisms are enhanced by adaptive responses (antibodies activate complement and opsonize bacteria for phagocytosis), while adaptive responses harness innate effectors (e.g. T cells recruiting neutrophils and eosinophils). This continued activity means that blocking the innate response can also be of enormous value in chronic inflammatory diseases—where such pathways are aberrantly and persistently activated. We will revisit this idea in Chapter 7.

Chapter 3
Adaptive immunity: a voyage of (non-)self-discovery

A key question addressed in this chapter is how the immune system can respond to so many diverse threats—including viruses (e.g. the severe respiratory infections SARS and MERS Co-V) that we have never encountered previously as a species. This inherent diversity in the immune system can be explained by analysis of how the adaptive immune system is put together—in particular the receptors on B and T lymphocytes.

B cells and antibodies

B cells are lymphocytes that develop in the bone marrow and are able to secrete antibodies for immunologic protection. Antibodies are highly specialized proteins that are able to bind to a particular target (e.g. the outer coat of a bacterium or virus), known as an *antigen* or *epitope*. Following binding this can lead to blocking of infection (*neutralization*), activation of the complement system, and uptake by phagocytes. If the antigen is on the surface of a cell (say, an infected cell or a cancer cell), it can lead to the killing of that cell. A vast range of antibodies can be produced and this ability to create a broad repertoire is essential—defects in antibody development leave individuals at risk of infection from viruses and bacteria, and indeed from cancer as well. The huge breadth of the antibody repertoire stems from the mechanisms used to make antibodies, which, although encoded in the genome like all other genes, undergo some particular tricks to create diversity.

Antibody (or immunoglobulin) genes are not created as a single unit—if this were the case we would have to inherit a huge number of closely related genes, and even this would carry the risk that it would not cover an individual threat. What is done instead is to stitch genes together from smaller parts, each of which is itself diverse, but which create many more possibilities through various combinations (see Figure 8). Each antibody is made up of two chains, a heavy and a light chain, and it is typically the combination of these chains which provide the specificity—in other words, the particular capacity to bind one individual target, for example this year's influenza strain but not last year's. The most specific piece of the immunoglobulin heavy chain gene is stitched together (or *recombined*) within the genome of a given B cell, from three types

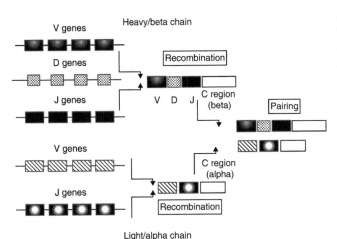

8. The DNA for an antigen receptor or antibody is made up of separate segments which are recombined. These are expressed as *heavy* and *light* chains, which pair together. The process of building a T cell receptor is analogous, except that *alpha* and *beta* chains are used.

of subunit—V, D, and J. Each of these is represented in the genome, side by side, multiple times (44 V, 27 D, and 6 J). Such segments can be combined more or less randomly to provide thousands of possible templates for antibody production. In fact, there is an additional level of diversity introduced as the joining process may introduce additional nucleotides (so-called *junctional diversification*), which can further modify the structure of the antibody at critical sites. A similar process, differing only in the lack of a D segment, occurs on the light chain. In humans, there are actually two different light chain genes, located in two different places in the genome.

Each B cell performs this recombining process independently, and thus as millions of B cells are made, they are able to explore fully the possibilities of combining heavy and light chains to create a very wide set of antibodies for host defence. The process of somatic recombination in B cells is regulated tightly by a number of genes—most importantly RAGs (recombination activating genes), which carefully control this somewhat dangerous process of manipulating and repairing host DNA. Loss of RAGs leaves the host without any means of creating such receptor diversity and thus with no adaptive immune system. Further modifications can be made later to antibodies to improve their effectiveness and 'bolt on' additional functions (see Chapter 4).

T cells: turning cells inside out

B cells create antibodies which can survey the extracellular environment—thus capturing viruses as they infect or spread between cells, or binding to bacteria which live outside of cells. B cells also possess a specific surface receptor, which is a membrane-bound version of the antibody it makes. By binding a soluble (i.e. free-floating) antigen, or a particle such as a virus, this receptor allows the B cell to receive signals about the presence of a target for its receptor. But viruses and other pathogens, including some parasites (e.g. the parasites that cause malaria) and bacteria (e.g. the TB-causing bacterium Mtb mentioned in Chapter 2), live within cells—so how can this internal environment be surveyed? This is the domain of the T cell and its specific sensor, the T cell receptor or TCR. T cells use a similar principle to B cells to create a receptor on their cell surface to interrogate the internal environment of cells.

The basic make-up of a standard-model T cell receptor is very similar to that of a B cell receptor (see Figure 8). The receptor is made of an alpha and beta chain, with similar genes making these up as are found in immunoglobulin heavy and light chains—that is, a palette of V, D, and J regions.

T cells need to sense the internal proteins of a cell—for example, a virus replicating within a target cell. To do this, the immune system has developed a pathway for revealing the protein contents of a cell on the cell surface (see Figure 9). All cells have a mechanism for degrading proteins via the *proteasome*, a complex of protein-cleaving enzymes which form a barrel-shaped organelle. Proteins targeted for degradation are decorated with a small molecule called *ubiquitin*, by a series of enzymes in a tightly regulated process. This includes any proteins made by an invading virus. The ubiquitin-labelled proteins are shuttled to the proteasome where they are cleaved into a variety of lengths of short amino acid sequences—*peptides* or *epitopes*—in the region of ten amino acids long. Such peptides are generated more or less randomly. Some of these peptides are actively pumped into the cell's export compartment, the endoplasmic reticulum, where they encounter the protein used to export them to the cell surface.

The protein used for export is highly evolved for this purpose and is encoded in a critical genetic area for the immune system known as the *Major Histocompatibility Complex* (MHC)—in humans also known as the *Human Leukocyte Antigen* (HLA) complex, or more commonly as the *tissue type*. HLA genes fall into two major classes, Class I and Class II, and in humans there are three major types

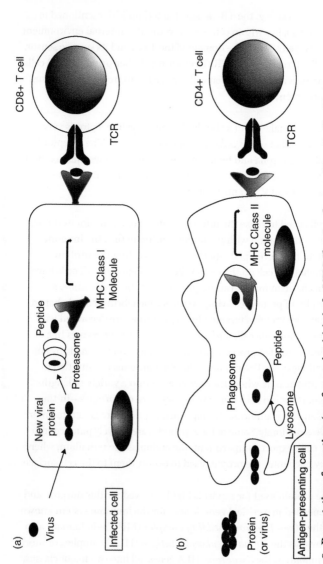

9. Presentation of an antigen (e.g. from a virus) (a) via the MHC Class I pathway to CD8+ T cells; (b) via the MHC Class II pathway, which is a feature of specialized antigen-presenting cells.

34

of Class I proteins: HLA-A, -B, and -C. Each of these molecules is highly adapted for carrying and presenting peptides—they possess a stalk for binding into the cell membrane and then a presenting platform in which there is a groove. Peptides are able to bind tightly into this groove. Thus a fully loaded HLA molecule will possess in its groove a single peptide, bound down tightly and 'visible' to the T cell. It is these peptides which are carefully sensed by the T cells through their receptors.

There is a vast array of possible viruses—and therefore peptides—thus the system of presentation through MHC has to be very flexible. Evolution has solved this problem through the creation of a huge array of different types (*alleles*) of HLA molecules. Across the globe there are more than 3,000 different types of HLA-A molecules and more than 4,000 HLA-B molecules found in humans, making it the most diverse region of the entire human genome. Unlike the B cell and T cell receptors, these do not recombine, and each individual only inherits six such Class I alleles (one set of HLA-A, -B, and -C from each parent). However, so diverse are these, and so many combinations exist, that very few of us have identically matching HLA molecules.

It is this huge diversity within HLA genes that creates a major issue for matching in the setting of organ or bone marrow transplantation, as in this setting, different HLA molecules coming in from the donor can be recognized as foreign, just like a virus, and induce a brisk immune response (see Chapter 6). Indeed, it was this property of providing a barrier to transplantation that first drew immunologists such as Peter Medawar to the MHC as a 'transplantation antigen' before its role in host defence was elucidated by Rolf Zinkernagel and Peter Doherty in the 1970s. The HLA region is the part of the human genome where the effect of evolution is most obvious—it is the most diverse. In other words, developing a wide range of HLAs has been essential for our survival as a species. The likely explanation for this is that it minimizes the chance of a microbe evading T cell responses and sweeping through an entire population. The problems faced by those looking to find matched donors for transplants are therefore a result of a successful evolutionary strategy for defence against severe infection.

Helpers and killers

T cells which are able to respond to peptides bound in the groove of an MHC Class I molecule are described as Class I restricted. They are also characterized by expression of the secondary receptor *CD8*. CD8 is not only a useful marker for these cells but actually adds to the specificity by also binding very weakly to the MHC molecule and stabilizing the interaction. Once a CD8+ T cell has recognized an infected cell, it is activated to proliferate (thus making more copies of itself and amplifying the response) but also to immediately respond to the threat by killing the target and releasing many signalling molecules—hence they are called *killer* or *cytotoxic* T cells.

There is another major type of T cell response which is involved in coordinating the immune response—the so-called T helper cells. These T cells are characterized by expression of the molecule CD4 on their cell surface and instead of sensing molecules presented by MHC Class I, they use a related system called MHC Class II, which is normally the preserve of a subset of immune cells called 'professional' antigen-presenting cells. The most effective of these cells is the dendritic cell, which has an unrivalled capacity to take up antigens derived from pathogens and present these to the immune system. Dendritic and related cells, such as macrophages, are able to take up, for example, a virus or bacteria, or a part of such a pathogen, into a specialized compartment known as a phagosome. The phagosome then fuses with an organelle called the lysosome. Lysosomal contents are highly acidic and so the pathogen is destroyed and broken down into peptides. These peptides are then immediately loaded onto a Class II molecule, which is then exported to the cell surface (see Figure 9).

Thus while B cells are able to sense and respond to the circulating threats (whole viruses for example), and CD8+ T cells to intracellular threats (viruses in a cell in a tissue), the CD4+ T helper cells sense what is provided for them by the professional antigen-presenting cells such as the dendritic cells. However, although this might appear somewhat limited, the role of CD4+ T cells is absolutely central to the functioning of the immune system, as is evident in the development of AIDS, where CD4+ T cells are lost as they are specifically targeted by HIV. The reason CD4+ T cells are so important is because they can provide help to both CD8+ T cells and B cells, and thus direct their activity. Since they receive their instructions from a highly specialized dendritic cell, they receive not only information about the antigens which are present, but also the context. As already discussed, dendritic cells will also sense the PAMPs associated with a particular infection and provide essential signals to the CD4+ T cell to direct its subsequent response. Since these instructions are given at the earliest stage of an immune response and the CD4+ T cells subsequently conduct the rest of the immunological orchestra as a result, this interaction, and the Class II molecules which direct it, have a major impact on host immunity and its regulation. There are number of different styles of helper T cell, distinguished by the different cytokines they make (e.g. Types 1, 2, and 17), which will be introduced in subsequent chapters as they have important roles in host defence, auto-immunity, and allergy.

Unconventional T cells

There are other T cells with different purposes that fill specific niches. These unconventional T cells differ not only in how they see antigens but also in their role in the immune response, since typically they are infrequently found in the blood but are very much present in the tissues. Here they also partly play the role of first responder seen in Chapter 2. The first such unconventional T cells identified were a T cell subset that, rather than using alpha and beta TCR chains, use a parallel set of receptor chains named gamma and delta, whose target is not the MHC. A series of molecules has been identified which can trigger gamma delta T cells—this includes a bacterial product HMBPP (4-Hydroxy-3-methyl-but-2-enyl pyrophosphate) which appears to function as a very potent ligand. It has been reported that a cell surface molecule, Butyrophilin 3A1, acts as a *presenting molecule* for gamma delta cells. Gamma delta cells are relatively uncommon in human blood but enriched at mucosal sites such as the gut and expand in response to bacterial infections. They are much more common in some other mammals such as sheep, where they may be the dominant type of T cell.

In addition to gamma delta T cells, there are alpha beta T cells with non-MHC specificities. Invariant NK T cells have, as the name suggests, some features of NK cells, but possess a TCR, although they emerge from the thymus with a uniform, distinctive alpha and beta chain. This receptor is able to bind a molecule that is MHC-like, named CD1d, which carries a glycolipid molecule

	Recognizes	Presenting molecule	T cell
	Peptide	MHC	Conventional T cell
	Bacterial metabolite (vitamin)	MR1 (MHC-like)	MAIT cell
	Bacterial metabolite	Butyrophilin	Gamma delta T cell
	Bacterial lipid	CD1d (MHC-like)	Natural killer T (NKT) cell
	Self-lipid in skin	CD1a (MHC-like)	Innate T cell

10. **An increasing number of unconventional T cell subsets have been found which recognize different types of molecules, some of which are similar to MHC molecules but usually not polymorphic (i.e. different between people).**

(i.e. fat- rather than protein-based recognition). One important molecule recognized by these cells is alpha galactosyl-ceramide, which has a combination of a sugar and a lipid molecule derived from bacteria. MAIT cells, mentioned in Chapter 2, are another example—these cells recognize the MHC-related molecule MR1, rather than MHC, presenting a vitamin B2 precursor made by bacteria (but not by humans). These and other unconventional or non-classical T cells are enriched in the liver and the epithelium of the gut in humans. There are likely many other T cell types with alternative recognition strategies to be discovered, probably providing host defence particularly at barrier sites (see Figure 10).

Distribution and recirculation

The lymphocyte subsets created through this process are not distributed randomly through the body but instead are carefully organized anatomically. Such organization is essential for mounting a rapid immune response, as we will discuss in Chapter 4. The CD4+ and CD8+ T cells which leave the thymus have a set of receptors on their surface which gives them specialized access to the lymphoid organs. This occurs through interaction with the blood vessel lining in these tissues organized into so-called high endothelial venules. In contrast they do not have access to normal tissues, even if they are inflamed or infected. The only exception to this rule is the liver, where the endothelium has gaps (*fenestrae* or windows) allowing direct contact between *naive* cells (i.e. cells that have not yet encountered a pathogen) and liver cell populations—a feature which may be relevant to the unique immunology of this organ (see Chapter 5).

Naive T cells can be found in the blood, recirculating between lymph nodes, and are highly concentrated in lymph nodes and the spleen. Naive B cells likewise are concentrated in these regions, which is critical for their biology as they require close interaction with T cells in order to develop into antibody-producing cells. T cells which have been activated are able to leave the lymph nodes, circulate through the blood, and relocate or *home* to tissues throughout the body, providing local defence. They do this by changing the receptors on their cell surface so they no longer bind to the high endothelial venule and instead are attracted to the inflamed endothelium. The unconventional T cells described earlier develop with this tissue-homing programme already in place so they are distributed to tissues directly. This makes sense, as their role is to provide immediate protection and they do not require further education and amplification in the lymph node.

Lymphatics are an important route for travel for lymphocytes as well as other immune cells. Lymphocytes leaving the lymph node do so via small lymphatics, which ultimately drain back into the blood system through the thoracic duct. Once in the blood the naive cells can then recirculate back to the lymph nodes, ensuring the whole range of B and T cell receptors, so carefully created, is well-distributed anatomically to counter diverse incoming threats.

In this chapter, we have seen how an immune system can be constructed to achieve a huge level of diversity from simple building blocks. The drive to do this is enormous—the MHC is the most highly diversified part of the human genome and has been under very strong selection pressure throughout human development. By maintaining a broad array of MHCs in a group, there is less chance of a pathogen overcoming the defences of an individual's or an entire population's immune system—the pathogen must tackle each person afresh. A failure to create MHC diversity would be catastrophic and could lead to an entire population being susceptible to infection.

The theme of diversity is continued and is even more obvious in the antigen receptors on B and T cells. Here the problem has been solved by evolution in a different way, using unique methods of recombination to effectively create millions of extra possible genes for this purpose. In the case of B cells, these genes, and the antibodies that are created from the genetic template, are further honed so they can become highly specific to their target. Effectively the genome of the B cell can be 'trained' to make the best immune response. Thus, while sensitivity and speed are the features of innate immunity discussed in the Chapter 2, diversification and specificity are the parallel features of the adaptive immune response discussed in this chapter. In Chapter 4, we will see how the immune response to such attack is coordinated, and how the potential diversity in attack is put to good use.

Chapter 4
Making memories

So far we have seen how the immune system can sense pathogens generally (e.g. via PAMPs and complement) and how it can target them specifically (e.g. via antibodies secreted from B cells and TCRs on T cells). Clearly all this needs to be tightly coordinated in space—to get the right cells in the right place—but crucially also over time. Let us consider how the response develops following exposure to a virus—following the dictum of Rolf Zinkernagel that viruses are the best teachers of immunology.

Priming the immune response

To make effective *memory*, the immune response needs to be induced correctly, or *primed*, during the initial stages of an infection. The first steps that must be taken by the immune system to develop a response relate to activation of the innate immune system. Without this, as has been established using genetically deficient mice, the adaptive response is subsequently overwhelmed in many cases. Indeed, HCV, which is able to establish chronic infection in most of those infected, is able to suppress and evade the innate immune response for many weeks in order to establish itself. Viruses which invade tissue locally are soon captured by myeloid cells such as macrophages and dendritic cells in order to initiate the innate response. Typically, a virus will present multiple PAMPs, leading to activation of these cells and kick-starting the process of antigen presentation.

Initiating this process in a tissue is of limited value if the aim is to allow presentation to a wide array of naive T cells in the hope of matchmaking the pathogen and its abundant peptide cargo with the appropriate TCR. The dendritic cell needs to relocate to the local lymph node, focusing on the areas where the T cells are concentrated. Here there is a very rapid series of interactions with putative responding T cells in an effort to find a match—in other words, a T cell that can recognize its cargo of MHC-bound peptides. As discussed in Chapter 3, a TCR likely exists for each possible peptide presented on an MHC molecule, although they may only represent one in a million of the normal pool of T cells, so this process must be very efficient, especially because at this point the race is on to develop an immune response as the virus is already replicating rapidly. This phase of the immune response is known as priming.

Once a T cell with the appropriate TCR is identified, the signals to that T cell are very potent and the changes within that cell are profound. One thing that must remain the same is the TCR itself, otherwise the specificity of the response will be lost. Therefore, with the aim of amplifying the response based on this recognition, the first response once such a signal is received is for the cell to proliferate, undergoing a process of cell division to create daughter cells. This proliferative response is enormous—within a few days the T cells responding to a single viral peptide may expand to represent one in ten of the CD8+ T cells in the body. It is also necessary—the T cells need to survey every tissue in the body to seek out and destroy virus-infected cells. The transformation in the T cell is very dramatic and in addition to proliferating, it rapidly acquires characteristics such as the ability to destroy the antigen; to make soluble molecules such as interferon gamma (which shares many antiviral characteristics with interferon alpha), tumor necrosis factor, and chemokines; and to attract other cells. Such cells are known as *effector T cells*, as opposed to the naive cells found pre-infection. CD4+ T cells are also activated and the populations of antiviral CD4+ T cells expand at this time.

Meanwhile a B cell response is also induced—again based in a lymph node. The organization of this B cell response is anatomically discrete—B cells secrete antibodies which can have an effect around the body even though the producing cells may be tightly localized. B cells require help from CD4+ T cells in order to produce fully optimized antibody responses. This activity is concentrated in specialized areas of the lymphoid tissue called *germinal centres* (see Figure 11). Within the sites where the antigen is concentrated B cells compete with each other for signals and space. This is a very effective way of ensuring that—from all the antibodies available—the most effective are amplified rapidly. Within the

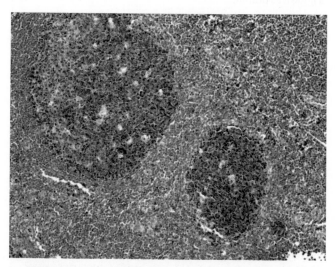

11. B cell responses are generated in germinal centres. These are illustrated as the discrete dark structures in this section of a tonsil.

germinal centre the B cells therefore undergo carefully coordinated rounds of proliferation.

The result of this is a surge in antibody-secreting B cells which eventually leave the lymph node and can be detected in the blood a week or so after an infection, accompanied by a rapid rise in antiviral antibodies. It is worth noting that not all antibodies directed against viral proteins are equal. Antibodies directed against the viral envelope proteins, which direct the attachment and infection of virus to host cells, are typically of the most protective value—although they are not always successful in neutralizing the target. If the virus is bound and recognized by the immune system in alternative ways (e.g. via complement) this may also provide some protection. Antibodies which bind a virus and prevent it infecting further cells are called *neutralizing antibodies*. Producing high levels of neutralizing antibodies is the goal of many vaccine strategies as this can provide complete protection against infection—a so-called *sterilizing immunity*.

The initial innate response and accompanying interferons, followed by rapidly emerging cellular (T cell) and humoral (B cell/antibody) immunity should reduce the number of productively infected cells and the spread of the virus between cells. This reduction in virus replication is important in the evolution of immunity since it means a reduced level of antigen and innate triggering. Here the B cell response and the T cell response diverge somewhat. B cells continue to mature and generate antibodies, and typically—after infection—these antibodies can be detected in the circulation for the rest of that person's life. Such antibodies are produced by B cells which have migrated to the bone marrow and actively secreted antibodies, having now become a specialized cell known as a *plasma cell*. T cells in contrast, are in the main much more short-lived. The response, as mentioned, expands very rapidly and *effector* CD8+ T cells reach very high numbers in the blood and tissues. In the absence of further stimulation, however, these cells die quickly and the population sharply contracts. This dynamic expansion and contraction makes sense in limiting the exposure of the body to very dangerous killer cells, which always have the potential to cause excessive tissue damage (i.e. *immunopathology*). However, this population is not lost altogether, persisting long-term as an immunological memory.

Laying down immunological memory

Immunological memory is considered the hallmark of adaptive immunity. It is on one level very simple—in fact it goes back to the definition of immunity in Chapter 1: immunological memory protects against a second exposure to the same infection. A person can be protected from a potentially fatal infection if the body has an immunological memory of the antigen. Such memory responses broadly work because the protective mediators (T cells, B cells, antibodies) are present in higher *quantities* and also possess appropriate *qualities* to fight a infection previously encountered infection. This combination of quantity and quality of these mediator cells means they can respond very quickly, leading to an absolute protection against infection, or at least a very rapid control and clearance of the infection before it has had time to establish itself or cause symptoms.

One of the most famous examples of memory induced by natural infection is that of an isolated Atlantic community in the Faroe Islands, who had been exposed to new infections only intermittently, through the arrival of seafarers. In 1846, the Danish physician Peter Panum went to the Faroes to investigate an outbreak of the measles virus—this virus has a very high attack rate in previously unexposed populations, with a high mortality rate in vulnerable groups (it killed one in five young children in an outbreak on the Pacific island of Rotuma in 1911). Panum noted that while the attack rate was indeed very high, a subset of individuals remained apparently uninfected—this was a group of elderly islanders who had been exposed to and survived a previous epidemic in 1781.

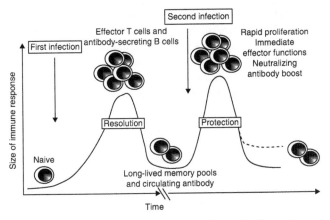

12. **After the effector phase, the large pools of B and T cells contract and memory is established. Upon re-encounter with the same infection these will re-expand more rapidly and also can reach higher levels in the bloodstream (termed *boosting*).**

Thus protective immunological memory established in one century had lasted half way through the next. It is very easy to imagine how such devastating infectious diseases could shape the evolution of the immune system (see Figure 12).

What processes underlie such long-lived protection? This question has long been debated by immunologists and continues to drive much interest in the field of vaccine research. Fortunately for the latter, a full understanding of this process has not been required in developing effective vaccines—simply harnessing the body's natural response to infection is enough in many cases. However, for complex infections such as HIV, looking under the bonnet of the memory response, taking the engine apart, and redesigning it will likely be required (see Chapter 7 for further discussion).

The best-understood part of the memory response, and broadly the most effective, is the induction of B cells and a very potent antibody that last for decades. B cells can improve the quality (stickiness or *affinity*) of their antibody over time. They do this by further adjusting the sequence of the immunoglobulin genes they originally made during the first few days of infection (see Chapter 3). The B cell of course does not know how to improve its antibody but takes the approach of an enthusiastic experimenter and attempts all available options in the hope of finding an antibody which works better. This process is controlled by a gene uniquely used by B cells—activation-induced cytosine deaminase (AID)—which deliberately mutates the relevant region of its immunoglobulin. AID works on an existing B cell response and helps improve the quality (affinity or stickiness) of the memory response (so called *affinity maturation*).

Memory antibody responses are also dominated by very active *IgG* antibodies that have a special additional quality which is that they cross the placenta. This is in contrast to the first antibodies that are made which are of *IgM* type (IgM antibodies are a good marker of there being an acute infection and are used for clinical diagnosis). One important consequence of this induction of strong IgG antibodies is that a mother's memory response can protect her unborn child against infection in utero. Beyond that it also is sufficiently long-lasting to continue to protect the newborn child. The level of transferred antibody drops in the baby over the first few months of life, but it serves to protect the baby effectively during his or her most vulnerable period. This added (perhaps *most* important) benefit happens naturally but could also be exploited further. For example, one interesting approach to vaccination against the virus Respiratory Syncitial Virus (RSV) currently being tested is to vaccinate pregnant women. This common disease is most severe in very young children and boosting maternal antibody levels is potentially a simple way of ensuring the youngest babies have sufficient protection at the time of greatest risk.

The B cell memory pool is organized in two parts—a set of *sleeper* memory cells, which reside in lymph nodes; and plasma cells, the highly differentiated set of B cells known as plasma cells (discussed earlier) which return to the bone marrow and are effectively antibody factories. This combination provides a balance within the immune system such that antibody-mediated protection can be sustained. Circulating specific antibodies provides immediate protection in neutralizing pathogens, and in some cases it is possible to infer the likelihood of successful protection by measuring the level of antibodies in the bloodstream (e.g. this test is done after vaccination against HBV to ensure a response has been made). The levels of these antibodies do however tend to wane over time after vaccination, and longer-term protection can be maintained by activation of the pool of memory B cells, which upon re-encountering the virus will rapidly proliferate and generate further antibody-secreting cells and high antibody levels. This means that even decades after an exposure, the system is primed to rapidly secrete further antibodies and provide effective protection.

T cell memory and its distribution

T cell memory is somewhat more complex since there is no simple marker like the antibody level equating to *protective immunity*. Nevertheless, we do understand the types of memory T cell that are induced and their likely roles in host defence, which is roughly parallel to those seen in B cells (this is true for both killer CD8+ and helper CD4+ T cells) (see Figure 13). Thus one set of T cells becomes the sleeper set, not actively functional but ready to respond in the case of re-exposure to the infection. These are located within lymph nodes and the spleen—ideal sites to re-encounter antigens if they are presented on an antigen-presenting cell (e.g. in the priming phase).

A second set of T cells has a more active lifestyle, homing in on peripheral tissues (such as the liver, gut, lung, etc.) and maintaining some elements of *effector functions* (killing capacity for CD8+ T cells and immediate secretion of specific cytokines).

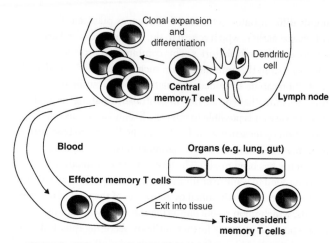

13. Central memory T cells are found enriched in lymph nodes. Effector memory cells are found in the bloodstream and enriched in peripheral organs. A further set of T cell memory cells are found resident in tissues.

These latter cells look in many ways like acute effector cells and have been termed *effector* memory in contrast with the sleeper cells found in lymph nodes which are termed *central* memory. Central memory cells, in response to an antigen previously encountered, will proliferate and acquire effector functions, homing in on tissues again, so the two populations are not independent of each other. In certain low-level chronic infections, such as CMV, the virus is never fully cleared, so there is a continuous activation of the memory pool and accompanying proliferation of these cells. The net result is that very large populations of effector memory CD8+ T cells can gradually accumulate in response to a single peptide, sometimes taking up about a third of the entire T cell memory population in the bloodstream (a process described as *memory inflation*).

In addition to these localization differences, there are other ways the T cell memory population can diversify, helping to tune the immune response against specific threats. For example, it has recently emerged that some populations of memory T cells found in tissues appear to have migrated there permanently—so-called *resident* memory cells. These may have a specific role in very early responses to infection in tissue, before it is fully established. Certainly overall, T cells play a distinct role in tissue defence and, unlike B cells which can act remotely via secreted antibodies, their immediate presence and local effector functions are required to protect the barrier surface.

Other T cells have developed a lifestyle focused on the germinal centre. T cell assistance in the germinal centre reaction is crucial in generating long-lived B cell memory. Vaccinologists have learned to harness this by attaching the target of interest to a specific protein which in turn attracts and activates these helper cells—a so-called *conjugate* vaccine. The newer vaccines against the pneumococcus (*Streptococcus pneumoniae*, the major cause of pneumonia in children and the elderly) are very effective and based on this principle. Further subtypes of T cell also can develop during such responses which have specialized properties. These include Type 2 cells, which are involved in defence against worms and also in allergy; and Type 17 cells, involved in defence against bacteria and yeasts. These will be dealt with in Chapters 5 and 6.

Harnessing B and T cell memories for immune protection

Having explored the mechanics of memory formation, let us consider how this has been harnessed in current vaccines and how this understanding may inform future vaccine development. The classic vaccines are called *live attenuated* vaccines, which are typically viruses that have been grown in tissue culture and have become less *virulent* (i.e. less able to cause disease) in the process. Vaccinia, the first vaccine used by Edward Jenner for protection against smallpox, is a related virus to smallpox but found as an infection in cows—it infects humans but causes a much milder and more limited disease. Since such vaccines are based upon viruses, they induce a response which mirrors that of a real infection, starting with recognition of innate triggers, antigen presentation, and induction of B and T cell responses to the presented antigens, followed by long-term memory formation. Providing the antigens are the same or largely shared between the vaccine and the real pathogen, a broad and protective response can be induced. This really is the ideal setting, as long-lived effective immunity can be readily generated—it may even be that since the pathogen is *live*, it may persist at tiny levels in specific niches, sufficient to keep subtly boosting the immune response in the long term. Such vaccines have provided protection against infections such as measles, influenza, and polio to countless populations, and vaccination has led to the eradication of smallpox (see Figure 14).

Another simple approach is to use a protein antigen. For example, this works well in inducing responses against the toxin in *Clostridium tetani*—an organism found in the soil which can

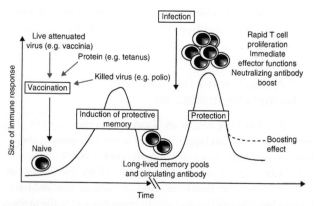

14. This figure shows the same process as described for memory following infection—only in this case it is induced by a vaccine. The same induction of memory T and B cells occurs, and these exert the same protective effects upon encountering the true infection.

infect wounds, leading to tetanus. Antibodies against the bacteria are not needed, simply the neutralization of the dangerous toxin, which is a protein. Administration of tetanus *toxoid*, where the protein toxin is inactivated by a simple treatment and made harmless, is followed by the induction of effective antibodies—and these block the activity of this highly potent toxin. A similar vaccine approach works against the toxin *Corynebacterium diphtheriae* (the bacterium which causes diphtheria). Both vaccines were developed in the 1920s by Ramon and Descombey and have remained virtually unchanged for nearly a century, saving countless lives over that time.

Protein antigens are typically administered with an *adjuvant*—a substance which causes non-specific inflammation and so enhances immunity. One such commonly used adjuvant is alum (aluminium salts), which can activate various innate pathways, although perhaps in future specifically designed adjuvants may become available, taking advantage of our new knowledge about the pathways that are necessary for full priming of B and T cells. They also generally need boosting, as the protein can be readily cleared, and repeated exposure is needed to drive the B cells through the germinal centre reactions required for expansion, affinity maturation, and class switching. Also such vaccines typically require boosting at a later interval, as the levels of antibodies tend to drop and further memory pools and plasma cells are required to sustain this. However, despite these limitations, protein-based vaccines to induce antibodies are hugely effective. Similar progress has been made using inactivated versions of whole viruses—for example, Louis Pasteur's rabies vaccine, which protects completely against a disease which is otherwise universally fatal.

Vaccines against bacteria such as Mtb (see Chapters 2 and 3), which live inside the cell and so would not be affected by antibodies or B cells, are much harder to develop—but there are several major targets. The oldest of these vaccines—and the only one licensed—is BCG, which is a live attenuated form of Mtb, which infects about two billion people globally. BCG (Bacille Calmette-Guérin), which was developed at the Pasteur Institute, has lost significant portions of its genome and is consequently highly *attenuated*. This vaccine has been trialled in many countries and can provide effective protection for children—a group in whom the disease can be very severe. However, its efficacy in adults is much less clear. Mtb sets up an intracellular infection just like viruses, so T cell-mediated immunity is important in its clearance. However, unlike antibodies, where it is possible to assign a protective function to a certain level of specific antibodies in the blood, defining what would be a protective level of immunity against Mtb and which of the many proteins it should possess as the best target is not straightforward. The task is made somewhat harder as Mtb shares antigens with harmless mycobacteria, which we are all exposed to, and which might influence the response to BCG (or newer vaccines) in later life.

One utility of immunological memory that has been harnessed for human benefit is the ability to transfer immunity from one person to another—so-called *passive immunity*. This was alluded to in the context of the transmission of antibodies from mother to child, where it happens naturally, but antibodies can be purified or concentrated for clinical use. One example of such treatment is to replace missing memory in individuals who lack the capacity to induce their own immunoglobulins. Simply transferring immunoglobulins of broad specificities at regular intervals can protect these individuals against serious infections. Such passive immunization has been used by doctors for many years in specific cases—for example, potent antisera can be used to protect individuals who are not immune but have been exposed to HBV, chickenpox (in cases where they are immunosuppressed or pregnant), or rabies. It can also be used after a snake bite to neutralize venom. The development of highly targeted monoclonal antibodies of a single specificity has huge potential in this area (see also Chapter 7).

The idea of memory in this context has long fascinated immunologists and neuroscientists alike. In both cases the development of a long-lived 'imprint' of an event is through a complex, multi-cellular system where the information is not stored or retrieved at a single site. Even if it is possible to identify lymphocytes we label as 'memory', they only act as part of a much larger team. In both cases, an element of rehearsal serves to fix the memory in the system—repetitive antigen stimulation or long-lived infections have an enormous impact in moulding the memory state. In both cases it even appears that false memories can be created—this is a natural by-product of cross-reactivity in the immune system. The consequences of such false memory in the shape of auto-immunity is dealt with in Chapter 6. Developing memories in advance, or 'getting your retaliation in first' to quote a British Lions rugby coach, through vaccines, has saved countless lives since the time of Jenner, and has the potential to save many more in the face of emerging infectious threats.

Chapter 5
Too little immunity: immunological failure

The immune system functions so well that most of the time we do not notice it is actually working at all. However, it is continuously active, preventing severe infection from the micro-organisms which colonize our skin and our gut, and suppressing the chronic virus infections most of us picked up as infants. In certain individuals, or under certain conditions, the immune response may, however, fail and this can lead to severe disease, the exact disease depending on the precise mechanism of failure. In this chapter we will examine how such failures may occur—specifically through genetic changes and through HIV infection—and also what we may learn from them about the working of the normal immune system.

Redundancy, polymorphisms, and knockouts

The immune system is a complex machine with multiple parts. In an ideal situation, every part functions perfectly, with induction of appropriate levels of immunity against commensal bacteria (i.e. not too much) and robust defence against infectious threats (i.e. just enough). If certain aspects fail, a number of outcomes are possible—in the same way as failing parts of a car have different impacts. One quite reasonable outcome is that nothing at all happens. For such a critical system there is apparently some inbuilt redundancy. For example, humans have multiple forms of interferon alpha, all of which do more or less the same job (i.e. protect cells against virus infection). One of the critical entry receptors for HIV is a molecule called CCR5, which is a chemokine receptor giving T cells information about where to traffic. Although the molecule is widespread, inherited deficiency of CCR5 has minimal impact on the health of the host, although as we will discuss later it has a huge impact on HIV infection. Losing some molecules is perhaps analogous to losing the spare tyre—not noticeable as long as the other four tyres are okay.

Other genetic defects have an enormous impact. Loss of the so-called *common gamma chain*, which is critical to the signalling of a number of molecules essential for lymphocyte growth and survival, leads to the development of severe combined immunodeficiency. Under these conditions most lymphocyte subsets simply fail to develop normally and the affected host is highly immunosuppressed. Another example was discussed in Chapter 1, where the thymus fails to develop in DiGeorge's syndrome, leading to a catastrophic failure of T cell immunity. This sort of defect is comparable to a large hole in the petrol tank—the car simply cannot run even if the rest of the machinery is intact.

There are a large number of other defects in the immune system—or subtle differences between people (genetic polymorphisms)—that have a more specific effect on immune defence. Loss of particular innate signalling genes can yield susceptibility to a narrow range of infections (such as rare viral infections of the brain). Mutations in a specific set of interferon genes (interferon lambda 3 and 4) can affect the rate of clearance of HCV and also the response to therapy—but apparently little else. They are perhaps, to continue the car analogy, more like losing a nearside mirror—most of the time this might not be noticeable but there will be a specific blind spot affecting particular manoeuvres. These specific relationships are of particular interest as they can tell us a lot about the bespoke requirements needed to protect against individual infectious threats, and how the immune system has evolved to deal with them.

Considering the differences between us that might influence the quality of immune responses (small differences known as genetic *polymorphisms*), the most important area of the human genome is the MHC, responsible for what is known as *tissue type* or HLA-type (see Figure 15). As discussed in Chapter 3, these molecules are responsible for presenting peptide fragments derived from pathogens to TCRs on T cells. Only those parts of a virus where the peptides can be bound into the groove of the MHC molecule are actually visible to the cellular immune system—T cells are more or less blind to the other parts. It is as if the MHC molecules need to reveal the information given by the virus, the rest being hidden.

The MHC is the most diverse part of the human genome—it has undergone intense selection over time, leading to a huge diversity

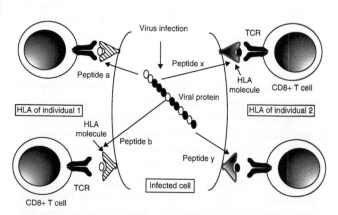

15. Individual 1 has a set of HLA molecules that, upon infection with a virus, may present peptides a and b; while individual 2 will present peptides x and y. In effect, their immune systems are 'seeing' the same virus quite differently.

of MHC molecules in the human population. Thus individuals'
MHC molecules vary quite widely in terms of the peptides they
select for presentation—and this can make a very big difference to
the immune response which is made. In other words, although
two individuals may be infected at the same time with exactly the
same virus, the peptides presented to their T cells may be entirely
different between the two people. In some situations this might
make no difference—all T cell responses might be equally good.
In others, however, the exact choice of peptide can be critical.
This is particularly the case in chronic virus infections such as
HIV and HCV. Here, peptide choice can be crucial. Certain MHC
molecules focus the immune response on areas of the virus
which are more effective targets, thus giving the T cells a relative
advantage. Those born with such favourable genetics have a better
outcome following infection (see HIV, discussed later in this
chapter). Similarly, there are unfavourable MHC types which
appear to direct a less effective immune response either because
of high variability in the viral peptide targets or even through lack
of such targets.

The ability to respond to a range of peptides is clearly crucial for
an individual to give them the best chance of finding a suitable
target on a virus. Across a population it is also an advantage
to have a diversity of such choice so that viruses cannot adapt to
escape responses generally. There are data to suggest that mate
choice (including in humans) can be driven by olfactory signals
derived from such MHC molecules—such that those with
divergent MHC types are chosen, hence maximizing the number
of different MHC molecules available to the offspring. Not all
animals are so lucky—in chicken colonies, where there is very
limited MHC choice, viruses such as Marek's disease have
succeeded in adapting to the host immunity in order to
enhance their infection. In humans, even though the range of
MHCs remains very wide, it is still observed that viruses such as
HIV may adapt over time across a population level to evade
recognition by MHCs and thus T cells. MHC molecules are in this

way said to leave their 'footprints' on the virus—but similarly through such intensive selection, viruses have left their footprints on the MHC too.

The MHC and the peptides it presents are so central to immune responses that MHC (or HLA) type is linked to a wide range of diseases (including auto-immunity, as will be seen in Chapter 6). However, it is not the only example where natural variation in human genetics can lead to weaker or stronger immune responses, even if the range is narrower. An important example is also seen in HCV infection, where it was identified that natural variation around the interferon lambda region was strongly linked to outcome of infection. In the case of infection with this virus, some individuals are able to clear infection spontaneously as a result of an effective immune response. With a particular mutation in the interferon lambda region this rate was increased around four to fivefold, and also increased the chance of successful clearance following treatment.

Interferon lambdas are a subset of interferons which share many of the same anti-infective properties as interferon alpha and beta already described, but which have a more limited tissue range—particularly working in tissues such as the liver and lung. The protective gene type is actually almost universal in some populations, so there may have been some selective force driving this—although it is to date unclear whether it impacts on any other infection. This is perhaps an example of a 'wing mirror' gene—critical for optimal function of the immune system but only in rather specific circumstances.

Inborn errors of the immune system

Some genetic changes lead to specific loss of a gene—a 'knockout'. These can also have rather pinpoint effects on the human immune system (see Figure 16). Although rare, such mutations can uncover a critical role for a specific pathway in control of certain

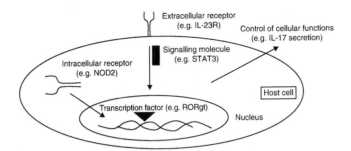

16. Defects in host defence can occur through mutations in cell surface receptors, signalling molecules, transcription factors, or effector molecules. Recognition molecules such as TLRs and NOD2 can impact on early events in immune activation.

infections. One example here would be loss of the Type 17 pathway, revealing a critical role for the pathway for the control of fungal infections. Individuals carrying mutations that affect this pathway, such as mutations in the extracellular receptor IL-23R, the signalling molecule STAT3, the master regulator transcription factor RORgt (which controls the cells using the Type 17 pathway), or in genes controlling cellular functions such as IL-17 secretion, suffer repeated and persistent fungal infections. This does not mean that the Type 17 pathway is only involved in fungal defence—experiments show that it is clearly involved in defending against bacteria as well—but it does indicate that its role in fungal defence is unique and cannot be performed by any other pathway.

Such human genetic data linked to human immune responses are very valuable but also very rare. In the last decades, enormous advances have been made by analysis of mouse models where specific defects have been engineered. The mouse immune system has been very well studied and many methods exist to examine the response to infection, tumours, and other diseases. To address the question of the role of a specific molecule it is now possible to introduce a genetic defect in a precisely targeted way into the mouse. This is a particularly powerful technique to define the role of a particular molecule, pathway, or cell type in either the normal immune system or in defence against a specific challenge.

Although advances in molecular biology have uncovered the basis for many of the defects which affect the immune system, many so-called *primary* (i.e. inborn) immune deficiencies remain to be fully defined. One relatively common group (around one in 50,000 births) is called *common variable immunodeficiency* (CVID). These individuals show a range of defects, most of which affect the ability to make effective antibody responses. Since the pathway to making an antibody is a long one, involving B cells and T cells cooperating around an antigen, a number of different defects affecting cell function and survival can lead to the same result. For those affected, they are susceptible to infection—most obviously, bacterial infections of the lungs. Repeated infections that are poorly controlled can lead to destructive lung damage (*bronchiectasis*), which in itself can badly impact on the normal immune defence system.

This clinical presentation does point to the critical role of antibodies in keeping control over the very common organisms that we all harbour such as *Streptococcus pneumoniae*. Other sites such as the gut, urinary tract, and eyes can also be affected—sites which can come into contact with bacteria regularly or continuously. Additionally, the immune dysregulation can be associated with auto-immune phenomena, indicating how finely balanced the system is under normal conditions. Fortunately, once it is diagnosed (which is not always straightforward, as it may take time to fully declare itself), treatment with transfusions of immunoglobulins from healthy donors can provide protection against the infectious complications of this disease. Since immunoglobulin levels decline with a half life of around three weeks, in the absence of a genetic cure, this therapy is regular and lifelong. It may be that with better molecular definition of the underlying causes in each case, alternative approaches to repair of the specific defects could be developed.

Malnutrition and immunodeficiency

At a global level, and throughout human history, an important cause of immunodeficiency is malnutrition. This can take a number of forms, including loss of specific micronutrients, such as vitamins and minerals, as well as protein-calorie malnutrition, which may well coexist. The exact impact of such malnutrition is variable depending on the function of the molecule—for example Vitamin D is involved in the development of regulatory T cells, while the Vitamin A pathway is involved in signals driving mucosal defence. T cells possess receptors for hormones involved in starvation. It has been shown that leptin, an important satiety hormone (i.e. one that suppresses appetite) can act not only on the brain but also to inhibit T cell function, providing a possible link between starvation (where leptin levels are high) and immune dysfunction. This is a complex area, where multiple different effects may overlap—worm infections, which are prevalent globally, can directly influence the immune system (see Chapter 6), as well as impacting on nutritional status and leading to iron loss, all of which could influence the response to infections with other micro-organisms.

HIV and Acquired Immunodeficiency Syndrome (AIDS)

How do pathogens exploit a normal immune system? One approach is to disable it, and this method is used by most viruses in order to create a specific niche or window of time in which to replicate. One virus above all has developed a strategy to exploit the immune system and turn it to its own advantage to devastating effect. HIV-1 (and its less prevalent relation HIV-2, found mainly in West Africa) is related to viruses found in many strains of African primates, including chimpanzees. It crossed over into human populations likely in the mid part of the 20th century. Like many viruses that cross species, it causes quite a different disease in each new host. Thus HIV relatives (so-called Simian Immunodeficiency Viruses or SIVs) can be carried in certain monkey species relatively harmlessly. This is probably a process of co-evolution, whereby the virus has adapted to the host to limit pathology and additionally the host populations have evolved to survive the infections. However, upon crossing species, the rules of engagement are rewritten and HIV-1 not only evades the human immune system but it also dismantles it (see Figure 17).

The first reason that HIV-1 is devastating to the immune system is because of the cell it targets for infection. HIV-1 uses two molecules in order to gain access to cells—CD4 and a chemokine receptor, typically CCR5. CD4 is the major molecule marking out T helper cells—it is the co-receptor for the MHC Class II molecules used for recognition by the T cell receptor. CCR5 is a receptor which allows the T cells to home in on sites of infection or inflammation, following cues laid down by other cells in the form of chemokine trails. Thus by using such receptors the virus is able to target T helper cells, particularly cells which have been recently activated. Infection of such cells can lead to a range of outcomes, none of which are good for the host. The cell may

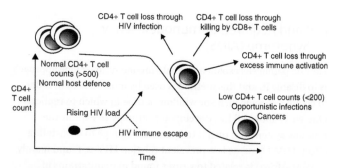

17. **CD4+ T cells are normally present at levels greater than 500 cells per microlitre of blood, but they fall as HIV infection progresses, which in turn is associated with rising viral load. Below 200 cells per microlitre the host is at high risk of opportunistic infections.**

become productively infected and generate more viruses. It may be recognized by the immune response and destroyed by CD8+ T cells. Or the virus may integrate and lay down a latent form for later reactivation.

The development of latency is a specific feature of the group of viruses to which HIV belongs—so-called retroviruses. These viruses are so-called as they are based as RNA, but can copy themselves back into DNA using a specific enzyme called *reverse transcriptase*. This DNA form of the virus is stable and is the template used to copy further versions of the virus genome and all the proteins required for virus function. It can be integrated into the host genome using a specific *integrase* enzyme which inserts the viral copy in among the host genetic material. If the virus is active, viral proteins will be generated and the cell will become a target for CD8+ T cells. However, if it is quiescent it will be invisible to the immune system and can persist as long as the cell (or its progeny) survives. This feature alone makes the virus very difficult to eliminate completely.

The infection of CD4+ T cells on its own would be a significant insult to the immune system if it resulted in a substantial loss of such cells—but if it were short-lived, it is likely such cells would recover rapidly. The fundamental problem with HIV is its ability to set up persistent infection, and thus the impact on the immune system is prolonged and extensive. How does HIV achieve this? One feature has already been mentioned—the development of a latent pool. However, while this represents real issues in terms of elimination in the long run, the persistence which occurs is associated with very high levels of virus in the bloodstream—thus active replication in the face of host immunity. One answer to this can be found by analysing the evolution of the virus within a host and observing the rapid adaptation to an individual host. The copying mechanism of HIV by reverse transcriptase has an interesting defect which means that the new copies are not 'proofread'. Thus each new copy of the virus contains at least one mutation. Given that there are trillions of copies of the virus generated daily and each contains around 10,000 base pairs in its genome, this means that every possible mutation it can make is potentially available to the virus. This huge pool of variants provides a rich resource for Darwinian selection, and this is exactly what is observed in the face of attack from B and T cells.

The antibody targets for HIV lie in the viral envelope—a difficult target since it is heavily *glycosylated* (i.e. coated in sugar molecules)—the molecules acting as a shield. Some of the most important and vulnerable areas are also hidden deeply and only open up on engagement with the cell to allow entry. Nevertheless, effective antibodies can be generated against HIV which should be able to neutralize and block infection by a given virus. However, single mutations in the virus genome can readily protect the virus against such antibodies and the development of such mutations in the envelope is exactly what is observed throughout infection. In other words, the immune system is able to control effectively any given virus strain through generation of antibodies, but the virus is able to remain one step ahead by generating new strains—the mutations often appearing to come at little cost to the virus.

So-called *broadly neutralizing antibodies* (bNABs), in other words, antibodies which could neutralize a very wide range of HIV mutants and so protect against infection, are a holy grail for HIV research. Indeed, these antibodies do develop after infection, but they take a long time to generate. If these could be generated using a simple vaccine approach, for example by focusing the immune response on the specific target from the start, this would be a huge breakthrough for the field.

The virus is, however, also under attack from the CD8+ T cell response and here additionally the ability to generate mutations gives the virus an advantage. Certain MHC types such as HLA-B27 and HLA-B57 are associated with better outcomes following HIV infection. A very rare group of patients who carry HIV are able to suppress it down to extremely low levels without suffering from progressive loss of CD4+ T cells. These so-called *elite controllers* are highly enriched for certain HLA types such as HLA-B27 and HLA-B57 (although other factors are also involved). These molecules bind peptides in the virus Gag protein, a molecule used to package the viral genome within the virus. Gag is relatively constrained in its ability to mutate compared to the viral envelope, and thus if the virus is forced to mutate to evade recognition by T cells, there may be a consequence for its Gag protein in terms of fitness. That is, every mutation that is made could subtly impact on the way that the protein functions, and so could impair the ability of the virus to replicate—a so-called *fitness cost*.

One way for the virus to manage this balancing act is to make multiple mutations to find a way of evading recognition while limiting the fitness cost. In such elite controllers therefore the virus is effectively pinned into a corner where it has a much more limited range of options to explore in terms of mutants and has already some compromise to its fitness. However, such outcomes are relatively rare. For the average person infected with HIV, the virus is able to mutate its T cell epitopes to escape the CD8+ T cell response and replicate effectively.

There are other factors which serve to limit the impact of the antiviral response and allow HIV not only to persist but to replicate to high levels. One is a specific down-regulation of the antiviral immune response referred to as exhaustion. This process occurs under settings where an immune response is very prolonged and is accompanied by up-regulation of off switches or checkpoints. The most well-known of these is *PD-1* (programmed death 1) which is able to limit T cell functions when it engages with its target, PD-1 ligand. This process is certainly active during prolonged HIV infection, and expression of a range of checkpoint molecules associated with the exhausted phenotype is linked to failure to control the virus. In the mouse model of LCMV (Lymphocytic Choriomeningitis Virus), where a similar process occurs during persistent infection, blockade of PD-1 can rejuvenate the T cell response and is associated with virus control. Such approaches are a potential avenue in infectious disease but have been much more influential in cancer therapies. Ultimately 'exhausted' T cell populations may simply be lost—or deleted. In HIV, it is not clear to what extent the T cell responses are truly exhausted, but any regulation of the immune response which limits the ability of CD8+ T cells to eliminate productively infected targets subtly shifts the balance of power in favour of the pathogen within the cell.

Although escape and exhaustion play an important role in allowing HIV to persist, this does not fully explain the massive loss of CD4+ T cells seen in HIV. Only a relatively small fraction of CD4+ T cells may be infected with the virus, but the impact is seen across the entire population. One explanation for this amplified effect is the development of *immune activation*: T cells which have been activated express certain surface markers such as HLA Class II molecules, allowing them to be tracked. The magnitude of general immune activation in HIV has long been found to indicate a worse outcome. It is likely that activated immune cells undergo more rapid turnover and death, and they are also more susceptible to HIV infection.

One of the prevailing theories for why immune activation may occur is that early in infection there is substantial infection of the CD4+ T cells in the gut. Normally these cells play an important role in barrier defence, and loss of such a barrier may lead to very low-grade transit of bacteria from the gut into the bloodstream (so-called *bacterial translocation*). Although this is insufficient to cause major infection, it is sufficient to activate the innate sensors in the immune system and trigger T cell activation. The long-term consequences of very early T cell infection in the gut may therefore be via this very indirect mechanism, although other innate responses to the virus itself may also contribute. Of relevance to this argument, the monkey strains which harbour

SIV without any harm (such as Sooty Mangabeys) show very low levels of such immune activation, despite carrying high levels of virus.

HIV infection therefore leads to loss of CD4+ T cells through direct infection, immune-mediated killing, indirect effects of immune activation, and likely many other mechanisms. HIV also can infect macrophages in tissues (which express low levels of CD4) and dendritic cells, and there are indirect effects leading to depletion of other cell types such as MAIT cells. However, of all of these the CD4+ T cell count in the blood is the best measure for the progression of the infection and the patient's risk of disease. The lower this drops, the greater the susceptibility to a range of pathogens, many of which are so-called *opportunistic*.

Even healthy persons are susceptible to TB infection, but the requirement for a fully intact cellular immune response to provide defence against TB means that, even relatively early on, the risk of disease is markedly increased. In contrast, there are a number of related mycobacterial infections which are never seen in a healthy immune system but become increasingly prevalent at low CD4+ T cell counts. At such low counts (<200 cells per cubic millimetre, where a normal count is >500) the patients are susceptible to a wide range of opportunistic infections including intracellular protozoan parasites such as *Toxoplasma gondii* (causing brain lesions), gut pathogens (e.g. *Cryptosporidium* species causing diarrhoea), yeasts, and fungi (e.g. *Pneumocystis jirovecii* causing pneumonia), and viruses such as the JC virus which can cause devastating destruction of brain tissue. These are all organisms which will be dealt with readily by a healthy immune system, but clearly these severe illnesses show the ongoing role of CD4+ T cells in coordinating that system.

One further disease category seen in such patients with acquired immunodeficiency is that of cancer. Two of the major cancers seen, Kaposi's sarcoma and B cell lymphomas, are driven by different viruses (HHV-8 and Epstein–Barr Virus or EBV, respectively). These viruses are both from the same group and are normally hard to eliminate in healthy individuals (EBV is a very common infection), but they are usually well controlled and cause little harm long-term. Uncontrolled replication is linked to the transformation of normal cells into cancer cells—thus such virally driven cancers are further examples of the central role of CD4+ T cells in controlling normal host defence against common antigens.

HIV is a devastating infection and—for the reasons described in this chapter—we still lack an effective vaccine. However, drug treatments are very effective at suppressing virus replication and halting the progression of the disease. Restoration of CD4+ T cell counts is, largely, associated with recovery of immune function and protection against opportunistic infections and cancers. Nevertheless, treatment is only suppressive—thus therapy must be taken lifelong with only one reported case of a person attaining a complete cure. This is one individual who has received a bone marrow transplant to treat a blood cancer, and in this transplant the marrow was from a donor who had a mutation in the CCR5 molecule. This mutation is relatively common and can influence the natural infection rate—if the person has two copies of the mutant gene this renders them highly resistant to HIV. The recipient of the transplant was able to effectively inherit this status with the donated marrow and subsequently has remained free of virus without further treatment. Unfortunately, so far, this individual remains the only example of such a cure.

This is a somewhat unusual and drastic therapy, but various attempts are being made to eliminate HIV from its long-term reservoirs in the body and provide an effective cure. As described earlier, the ability to lay down a latent pool gives the virus an enormous advantage over the host—the immune system is not able to visualize and respond to cells where the virus is not replicating, and drugs are equally inactive. One approach is to activate the virus using a range of approaches and then destroy the cells which have revealed their virus before they go on to spread it further. This is a complex area, since the actual site of the cells where the reservoir is located, their status, and the means to fully eliminate them are all poorly defined. As such, for the time being the main thrust must be to get as many people who need therapy onto an effective treatment and to stop the spread of infection by means of education and appropriate interventions (including pre-exposure treatment programmes). In the meantime, the search for an effective HIV vaccine continues.

Chapter 6
Too much immunity: auto-immunity and allergic diseases

Much of the emphasis so far in this book has been on providing defence against micro-organisms, and this is the major driving force for the evolution of the immune system. This is clear from the severe disease syndromes that occur when the immune system is deficient (seen Chapter 5). However, given the capacity to cause tissue damage and inflammation, every immune response must be appropriately and specifically tuned. Failure to tune in appropriately leads to a range of immunologically driven diseases that, given the general improvements in health status and many major infections in Western populations, have taken on increasing significance. In this chapter we will address how the immune system acts to turn off unwanted responses, and what goes wrong when this fails. This includes looking not only at classical auto-immune diseases but also at other diseases where there is excessive inflammation. It also includes consideration of allergic diseases, where there is an exaggerated response to harmless antigens, dominated by a particular style of immunity.

Tolerance in the thymus

To understand how auto-immune diseases occur it is important to review how the immune system takes steps to avoid this—by so-called *immune tolerance*. The rules are somewhat different for T and B cells, but since CD4+ T cells are crucial for the development of most long-lived antibody responses, if the T cells are well controlled then the B cell compartment will follow. T cells are educated primarily in the thymus, so this is the most critical site where self-tolerance is learned.

One puzzle for T cells is how to ensure the TCRs that are generated are of any use. Since the T cell puts the TCR together at random and the recognition of an antigen is completely dependent on the MHC molecules present in that individual, it is likely that many TCRs are of no value in an immune response. This is not the case for B cells, where the antigen could be very broad—a protein, a sugar molecule, a lipid (fat), or even a chemical. The problem is solved by providing some early education for the T cells in the thymus. Two essential processes take place in the thymus—so-called *positive* and *negative* selection (see Figure 18). Positive selection is a process to ensure that the repertoire has some ability to recognize

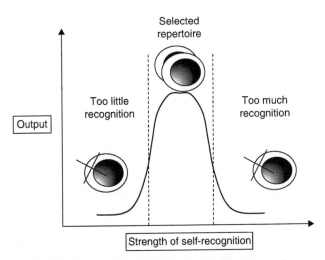

18. The T cell (CD4+ or CD8+) will encounter self-antigens as it develops in the thymus. Those T cells where such interactions are too strong or too weak are eliminated (i.e. central tolerance).

self-MHC—in other words, the particular suite of MHC molecules present in that person.

Upon entry into the thymus as a very early and immature cell, the T cells start to arrange their T cell receptors. As we discussed in Chapter 3, there is a huge range available; what is required are receptors which are able to engage with the person's own MHC molecules but not react against self. This is an interesting balancing act as no pathogens are available in the thymus of a developing foetus or newborn child on which to base this choice of self versus non-self. The way the immune system solves this problem is to present a wide range of self-peptides in the thymus through the activity of a specific gene called *AIRE*. This allows the cells in the thymus to make proteins normally made only in very specialized cells in the body (e.g. from the pancreas or brain) and then eliminate T cells which react against these. Similarly, T cells which completely fail to engage with the self-MHC are also eliminated. Only those in a narrow 'Goldilocks range' of recognition—just enough but not too much—are able to exit the thymus and form the naive pool.

This is a really crucial step in immunological education, as evidenced by the impact of genetic loss of the AIRE gene and the consequent disease caused by the induction of auto-reactive T cells and antibodies. AIRE is a highly specialized molecule which allows the thymic cells to express molecules normally only restricted to specific tissues—insulin, for example, which is normally made only in the pancreas. The loss of AIRE through mutation therefore allows a range of T cells to escape the thymus that would otherwise normally be eliminated, and leaves the individuals (who are very rare) prone to auto-immunity. In particular, they suffer from reactivity against their own glands (e.g. the thyroid and parathyroid glands). As an apparent paradox they may also suffer from increased susceptibility to yeast infections—but this is due to antibodies fighting their own cytokine Interleukin 17. As we saw in Chapter 5, Interleukin 17 is crucial in defence against surface Candida infections, so this combination of auto-immunity and immunodeficiency is the result of the same process of lack of self-tolerance.

Peripheral tolerance

However, even if AIRE is fully functional, this process is still not sufficient to protect fully against auto-immunity, and a 'belt and braces' approach is taken by the immune system. Tolerance can be broken, for example, if a rogue T cell escapes the thymus without having been properly educated, or if there is very close mimicry between a pathogen and a self-protein. This may sound unlikely, but what is actually recognized by the T cell receptor is a short peptide, which is bound in the MHC groove and presents perhaps only two to three major amino acids that are recognized. Thus even if the peptides themselves differ between, say, a virus and a protein from the brain, by the time it has been bound and presented in the MHC, the overall shape recognized may overlap somewhat. The thymic system thus must be flexible enough to allow T cells to escape where such cross-reactivity may exist, otherwise the ability to respond to pathogens would be excessively limited. In other words, it is somewhat leaky—or the immune system needs to take a small risk in releasing T cells.

But if rogue (or potentially rogue) T cells are circulating in all of us, why do we not all succumb to auto-immunity? One possibility is just ignorance. If antigens are hidden away, and therefore not presented to the immune system on an antigen-presenting cell such as a dendritic cell (by the processes described in Chapter 3), the immune response will never be triggered. This phenomenon may account for lack of responsiveness to specific tissues such as the brain, which is protected by the blood–brain barrier, a physical barrier that largely excludes cells of the immune system from entering the brain. However, in experimental models it is still possible to induce auto-reactivity against the brain by vaccination with brain-derived proteins or peptides—such peripherally induced cells are able to cross into the brain and cause disease, so such a 'Maginot line'-style defence is not adequate for complete protection.

Tissues also protect themselves. Some possess mechanisms to down-regulate T cells—for example, they may express death receptors (Fas-ligand) which engage molecules on T cells to kill them. PD-1, which we discussed previously in the context of immune exhaustion, is also an important off-signal for T cells. Mice that lack PD-1 are highly prone to auto-immune disease. This is a very interesting example whereby viruses have essentially harnessed an off switch present in the immune system to down-regulate immune responses and allow them to persist. Another similar inhibitory molecule is called CTLA4. CTLA4 is expressed on T cells and binds the same molecules as an activatory receptor called CD28. CD28 triggering is very important in the initiation of immune responses—but CTLA4 can interfere with this and abrogate such reactivity. Mutations leading to loss of CTLA4 lead to severe auto-immune disease, with marked proliferation of lymphocytes. Interestingly, CTLA4 possesses a number of variants in the population and certain variants are strongly linked to auto-immune disease of the liver, thyroid, pancreas (causing diabetes mellitus), and gut. These variants can be posited to tune the immune reactivity of the host, and in combination with other similarly subtle defects can contribute to the development of clinical auto-immune syndromes.

As we learned in Chapter 5, rare inherited diseases can beautifully illustrate the importance of specific cells or pathways, and IPEX syndrome is one such example. Here there is loss of FOXP3, a molecule which is essential for the development of a set of T cells described as T regulatory cells or *Tregs*. Loss of Tregs is associated with severe auto-immunity and these cells clearly play an important role in maintenance of a healthy, steady state in all of us. Tregs can be derived via a number of routes, and have a range of specificities—but they are all able to act on other immune cells, notably other T cells, to inhibit their proliferation and many other functions. Some Tregs are actually derived from the thymus—rather than deleting auto-reactive cells the thymus actually turns them to good use by inducing a regulatory programme. These Tregs exit the thymus and can help to control auto-reactivity through the release of inhibitory cytokines such as Interleukin 10 and Tissue Growth Factor beta (TGFb). They also express high levels of the Interleukin 2 (IL-2) receptor CD25—a molecule used as an important surface marker for such cells. Interleukin 2 will be sensed by Tregs even at low levels and enhances their function—when auto-reactive T cells are activated IL-2 is made, and this can enhance Treg activity and limit auto-immune disease.

Because of the way T cells are sequentially selected in the thymus, if a self-reactive T cell is generated against a specific target, a Treg will be similarly generated to essentially keep an eye on it in the periphery. However, if needed, Tregs may also be induced in the periphery from otherwise standard T cells—these also develop through expression of FOXP3 and development of regulatory activity and upregulation of the IL-2 receptor. The situation can be somewhat complex, however. Depending on their origin, T cells may possess both pro-inflammatory and regulatory activity. Although this is somewhat confusing for immunologists trying to neatly organize cell types, it is clearly an advantage for the system to have sufficient plasticity that T cells can modulate their function as the situation develops.

One further mechanism of tolerance to be considered comes from the emergence of the *danger theory* of Polly Matzinger, or the infectious non-self model of Charles Janeway. Both of these theories considered that the important issue about whether an immune response was made against an antigen was not whether it was self or non-self, but *how* it was presented to the immune system. Antigens which are presented in the context of inflammation or infection (i.e. in a dangerous situation) will induce a response—but the same antigen presented in the absence of such signals will not. Immunologists have intuitively understood this for decades as they have made use of *adjuvants* (often bacterial products) in order to induce effective responses to vaccines. This now makes molecular sense as we understand much more about how such danger signals or PAMPs are sensed by the immune system and their impact on the antigen-presenting cell, as discussed in Chapter 2. It also makes sense given we now understand that the process of self-tolerance in the thymus is imperfect so many other layers of protection must be afforded. One interesting, but fortunately rare, cause of auto-immunity is dysfunction of innate immunity in the disease Aicardi–Goutières Syndrome. Here there is failure to break down DNA effectively—so when cells die naturally their DNA is not disposed of appropriately. Free DNA within a cell is recognized as a danger signal through the pattern recognition receptor CGAS (see Chapter 2) and so this genetic defect leads to an enormous level of innate response—as if there were an ongoing virus infection. The ongoing inflammation induces auto-immunity, tissue damage, and severe disability in those affected.

The take-home message is that in the absence of innate signalling resulting from a pathogen or inflammation, an antigen should be ignored, whether it be self or non-self. This is an important scenario, as a self-reactive T cell sitting, for example, in a lymph node could very well receive signals through its TCR if its antigen is carried to it on a dendritic cell from a local tissue. If the dendritic cell has not received any signals regarding infection or inflammation, then the signal is safe, and the consequence is a phenomenon described as *anergy*—that is, loss of reactivity to further stimulation. Anergy leads to a failure to respond to future signals, and results from receiving only a TCR signal without accompanying co-stimulation or cytokines. It is a further, effective way to very specifically control auto-reactive cells in the periphery. Providing only partial signals to T cells is also a trick played by pathogens. HBV and HCV, for example, are viruses which induce an extremely poor innate response—thus although there is plenty

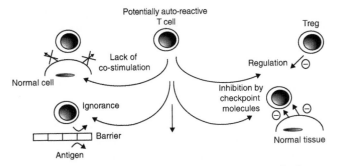

19. A number of different and overlapping mechanisms may lead to suppression of function or physical elimination of potentially auto-reactive T cells which have emerged from the thymus (i.e. peripheral tolerance).

of antigen presented to the immune system, responses cannot be properly initiated and it may take months to induce an effective T cell response. The mechanisms involved in peripheral tolerance are summarized in Figure 19.

Tolerance in specific organs: the liver and the placenta

The viruses HBV and HCV, mentioned earlier, also have a distinctive feature of targeting the liver, and it is no coincidence that they are able to set up long-term infections in this organ, as its immunologic profile is quite distinct from other tissues. The most striking data on this come from the work of Roy Calne in the 1960s, who developed a programme of liver transplantation in Cambridge. His work, described in the *Lancet* editorial 'Strange English Pigs', showed how transplantation without rejection was possible across conventional transplantation barriers. To understand the significance of this, it is first necessary to understand an important issue in transplantation of organs.

For other organs (e.g. kidney, heart, pancreas, and lung) there must be accurate matching between the recipient's MHC molecules and the donor's, otherwise there is a vigorous immune response. Although at first sight this may appear unexpected as the host's T cells are trained to recognize their own MHC molecules, it turns out that a foreign MHC presenting even an innocuous peptide will be bound and recognized as if it were a virus. In other words the overall shape of the foreign MHC is sufficient to engage T cell receptors and trigger an immune response. This response is further increased since graft will be put in through surgery, causing tissue damage and alerting the immune system through innate inflammatory responses. Thus in the normal case, if MHC matching between the donor and recipient does not occur, many T cells can be mobilized that home in on the graft, which causes major tissue damage and the graft to be rapidly rejected.

In the liver, however, MHC matching is not required. Furthermore, the recipients who have successfully engrafted a liver can also receive other organs from the same donor. In other words the liver graft has made them specifically tolerant to certain foreign antigens—the graft does not make them generally tolerant, only to the MHC molecules in the donor. In human liver transplants the same occurs—matching of donor recipient is only required in terms of blood type, and eventually the acceptance is so complete that in some cases no immune suppressive drugs are needed.

It is not clear exactly how the liver achieves this feat, but one mechanism is to present antigens with very limited co-stimulation. T cells which detect antigens under such circumstances fail to proliferate effectively and will undergo premature death. The liver contains its own specialist set of antigen-presenting cells in the form of liver sinusoidal endothelial cells which can avidly take up and present antigen. In the absence of inflammation these can effectively tolerize immune responses. Since the liver's blood supply is vast, and the cells move very slowly within the organ, these interactions are quite frequent and efficient.

One other interesting feature of the liver is that the endothelium is *fenestrated* (i.e. it has gaps or windows that allow the lymphocytes within the blood to contact the tissue cells—normally they would have to traverse the endothelium in order to do this). This feature means that naive T cells which do not possess the homing receptors that would allow them to enter tissue can potentially detect antigens presented in this organ. Efficient priming of the immune response normally occurs in the lymphoid organs, where it is supported by the correct blend of dendritic cells, co-stimulatory molecules, cytokines, and stromal support. The encounter of antigens for the first time in a peripheral tissue is likely to lead to partial and therefore ineffective activation as described earlier.

Why would the liver be designed this way? One argument is that we need to be tolerant to our own microbes living in the gut and the antigens from the food we eat. Since all the blood supply from the gut drains through the liver, presenting antigens in this *tolerizing* environment is one way to limit responses. Clearly this needs to be finely balanced since if a significant invasive pathogen comes via this route it is an ideal place to stop its spread before it reaches the rest of the body, and indeed the liver possesses an array of antimicrobial defences which are necessary to limit such spread—particularly an effective set of tissue-resident macrophages (Kupffer cells) which can engulf microbes. However, overall it appears the system is quite heavily regulated or dampened—the hepatitis viruses mentioned earlier clearly exploit this tolerant environment in order to establish viral persistence.

A further environment where it is essential to damp down immune responses which will naturally occur is in the setting of pregnancy. The foetus and placenta contain antigens which belong to both the mother and the father—unless the two are very closely related it really represents a mismatched graft and should be rejected. Clearly there is a set of tolerance mechanisms in place to prevent this occurring, including those described earlier. The entire immune system of the pregnant mother is in fact influenced by this process such that she is moderately immune-suppressed, and therefore at higher risk from certain infections such as varicella zoster (chickenpox) and malaria.

One interesting factor which can restrict immune responses in the placenta is modulation of immune metabolism. T cells require plentiful supplies of amino acids in order to function and one of these—tryptophan—can be seen to play an essential role, since specific loss of this molecule from their environment can turn off T cell activation. Restriction of tryptophan in the local environment is therefore a powerful way of arresting responses in the placenta, and this is done through up-regulation of an enzyme called indoleamine deoxygenase (IDO), which breaks it down effectively. IDO is not restricted to the placenta and indeed is activated in dendritic cells which allows them to regulate responses following activation. However, it has been shown that blocking IDO leads to immunological rejection of the foetus in mice, thus indicating it has an important role in foetal tolerance.

The liver has its own version of IDO (TDO) which is continuously generated and may serve to promote tolerance in that organ. Tryptophan is not the only amino acid manipulated in this way to modulate inflammation. Arginine is also essential and can be sequestered away from T cells to limit their function through the action of arginase, as found in tumours and in a specific group of regulatory cells related to macrophages described as myeloid suppressor cells.

Auto-immunity and inflammation

Having established the mechanisms which hold auto-immunity at bay, and having been introduced to some of the severe syndromes which occur if these fail, let us consider some common and complex auto-immune and inflammatory diseases. One of the best known of these is rheumatoid arthritis (RA), which leads to inflammation of the joints and ultimately their destruction, in severe cases, as well as being associated with inflammatory tissue damage to other organs. The cause of RA is not known, but let us consider one interesting hypothesis which pulls together many known strands.

The risk of RA is highly dependent on specific MHC molecules, particularly Class II molecules (such as HLA DRB1* 04). This indicates that presentation of specific peptides from these molecules is part of the cause of the disease. The disease is also clearly associated with the development of antibodies to a specific class of protein—*citrullinated* proteins. Citrulline is a modification of arginine which can occur during inflammation, for example, and by changing the shape of the antigenic protein it creates a new target for the immune system. Antibodies to citrullinated peptides are used as part of the diagnostic tests for RA. It is also seen very early, again suggesting it is linked to the cause of the disease. Smoking is also increasingly linked to RA—the risk of RA rises with both the duration and the intensity of smoking.

One idea therefore put forward by Lars Klareskog and colleagues is that smoking leads to the generation of citrullinated proteins which potentially form new targets for the immune response. In the presence of a *risk* HLA molecule, these new peptides are presented and tolerance is broken, followed by the development of antibodies to these modified targets. These auto-immune reactions can impact on both the lungs (which may show changes in RA, even if it is not clinically apparent) as well as the joints. It may be that a second hit is required to initiate the joint inflammation, since the antibodies can appear many years before the joint disease develops. Overall, this is an interesting idea which links the genetic and environmental factors driving RA, and also suggests that there are different variants of RA with different causes, since some individuals do not develop antibodies to citrullinated proteins. The factors involved in RA are summarized in Figure 20.

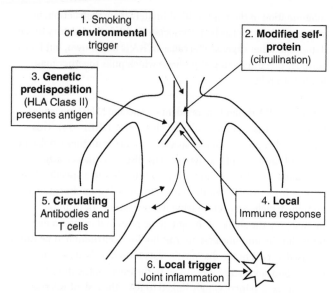

20. A model for rheumatoid arthritis (RA) proposed incorporates some of the known genetic and environmental triggers. The inflammation can also be linked to development of disease symptoms outside the joints (e.g. in the lung or skin).

Multiple sclerosis (MS) is a potentially devastating disease resulting from auto-immune responses occurring within the central nervous system. This inflammation leads to loss of the myelin sheath around nerves and thus loss of their function. It is typically an intermittent disease, with attacks, followed by a period of quiescence, but it can lead to cumulative disability over time. Like RA, it is also strongly linked to HLA Class II genes, in this case the DR2 complex (e.g. DRB1*1501), suggesting a role for T helper cells in its initiation. MS also has a very interesting connection between genetic and environmental causes. It is much more common in temperate climatic zones, such as northern Europe and the US (or early migration to those zones), much more common in women, and also increasingly linked to infection with EBV.

EBV is a very common infection throughout the globe, nearly ubiquitous in some settings, and MS is thought to occur in 2.5 million individuals, so it cannot be a simple relationship between cause and effect. One idea is that there is epitope mimicry between a peptide from EBV and one from the brain tissue (e.g. myelin basic protein)—this mimicry would only be seen when the peptide was presented by the risk MHC protein, explaining the genetic risk. Alternatively, EBV infection in the brain of a susceptible individual could reveal self-proteins to the immune response and break tolerance to self, by providing the necessary danger signals (as discussed earlier).

The latter idea may be extended by considering one explanation for the geography of this disease which relates to sunlight exposure. Lack of sunlight in regions away from the equator is linked to lower Vitamin D levels—this vitamin has an important regulatory role in the immune system, and low levels are associated with auto-immunity. Interestingly, genetic variants which affect the levels of Vitamin D made in the body have an impact on MS risk, strengthening this causative association. There are some complex interactions between sex hormones and the immune system, but lower testosterone levels may also influence overall immune reactivity and are also linked to enhanced MS disease progression.

Overall, a picture is emerging of a series of steps between initiation of inflammation in the brain and development of clinical disease—normally these can be well regulated through all the checkpoints described earlier, but a series of environmental and genetic risks can tip the balance in favour of disease if they accumulate unfavourably. Fortunately, by picking apart some of these genetic risks, the door is opened to potential new therapies (such as modulation of Vitamin D or sex hormone levels), in addition to the biologic agents that target the immune cell populations responsible, discussed in Chapter 7.

Another auto-immune disease with complex causes resulting from a gene–environment interaction is inflammatory bowel disease (IBD). IBD is in fact at least two diseases—Crohn's disease is associated with deep fissures in the bowel and can occur anywhere along the gastrointestinal tract (including, for example, the mouth as well as the small bowel), while ulcerative colitis can lead to very severe inflammation affecting the large bowel only. Both may in fact be associated with some inflammatory features outside the gut (in joints and skin, for example), and they share genetic risk factors with each other and with other auto-immune diseases of those organs (ankylosing spondylitis and psoriasis, respectively). This points to a common pathway for inflammation and possibly an overlapping causation.

While RA and MS affect organs where there is normally no microbial presence (sterile sites), IBD affects the gut, which is the home to trillions of bacteria as part of our normal gut flora or *microbiome*. A number of rare inherited genetic defects can lead to IBD. IL-10 is a cytokine which can powerfully suppress immune responses. Loss of this molecule or loss of its receptor and downstream signals leads to very early onset of the disease. These point to an important role for immune regulation in control of responses to the microbiome, and the prevailing model for IBD is that this fine balancing act breaks down, leading to continuing inflammation. The normal microbial content of the gut must be largely ignored by the immune system, even though if the same microbes moved only a few millimetres across the gut wall into the bloodstream they would represent a major health threat. There is likely a continuous process whereby any misplaced microbe is dealt with very efficiently without the need to activate a full inflammatory response—these aggressive responses are, however, readily brought into play if a real pathogen attempts invasion.

The genetics of IBD are very striking and point to two important strands leading to disease. First is the Type 17 defence axis which we encountered earlier in the context of surface defence against yeasts, and this is regulated by cytokines such as Interleukin 23 (IL-23). Variants in genes influencing this axis are linked to increased risk of IBD. Second, the innate immune response is also important, since a specific gene, NOD2, is involved and this is a pattern recognition receptor for bacteria. Failure to recognize and rapidly deal with relatively harmless *commensal* bacteria may promote ongoing immune responses in the gut and set up a vicious circle whereby gut damage leads to further exposure to bacteria in the host tissue (see Figure 21).

There are a number of interesting new approaches to suppressing such inflammation, for example specific blockade of cytokines and chemokines (discussed in Chapter 7 in more detail). The cause of the disease, however, is a poorly balanced relationship with one's own gut flora, and this has a much wider implication for human health.

Microbiome populations are very complex and only with new molecular techniques is it becoming possible to dissect out the

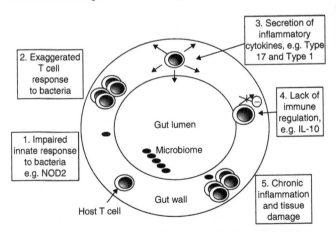

21. **Inflammatory bowel disease (IBD), Crohn's disease, and ulcerative colitis have a very strong genetic predisposition but also require an environmental trigger (likely the microbiome of the gut).**

vast array of species living within a single individual's gut. Many of these are not possible to culture with standard methods and have been ignored to date by microbiologists who naturally have focused on organisms that have been linked with disease. The relationship between host and microbiome has evolved over time as the flora are acquired after birth, and each individual will develop a slightly different balance. The flora also modulate the development of the immune response through exposure not only to PAMPs and bacterial antigens, but also to bacterial metabolic products, and this can have an important influence on the host immune response not only at the gut interface but also throughout the body.

This area of study has attracted a lot of attention recently, and different microbiome populations have been associated with different types of disease, from IBD, through RA and MS, to obesity, Parkinson's Disease, and Alzheimer's Disease. This type of research is still at a relatively early stage, so closely tying a specific change in a microbial population to a mechanism leading to a disease has been rarely achieved. However, if causality is proven, taking steps to modulate the gut microbiome may provide an interesting additional intervention to prevent or even treat a range of disorders. It should also be noted that the gut is not the only part of the body with its own microbiome—even within the gut this varies, but there are also bacterial commensals living in different regions of the skin and throat. These likely not only influence the local immune systems but have a potentially wider impact.

These three examples all show how different genetic and environmental triggers combine to increase the risk of auto-immune disease. Each individual risk may be relatively small, but the combination of risks serves to break down the security defences which have been set up through evolution to protect against auto-reactivity. One way of looking at this is that there are usually multiple layers of defence, and thus a number of things need to go wrong for auto-reactivity to cause problems. Given that the risks from each impact, genetic or environmental, tend to be rather small on their own, very large studies—usually of thousands of affected patients—are required to detect their effects. Fortunately, the genetic technologies and analysis of *big data* (huge stores of electronic health data) have reached a point where this is possible.

Allergy

Allergy is related to auto-immunity in the sense that it is a failure of the immune response to respond to normal cues, leading to an exaggerated and harmful response to inappropriate antigens. In this case the substance is not self, but it is harmless (non-dangerous) non-self. Through the mechanisms of tolerance described earlier, exposure to such an antigen, such as pollen, proteins from house dust mites, or food, should evoke minimal responsiveness. However, aberrant responses or hypersensitivity to such antigens is remarkably common and can be very dangerous.

The hallmark of allergy is the induction of a Type 2 immune response, driven by a specific set of T cells called Type 2 T cells (see Figure 22). Type 2 T cells tend to secrete lower levels of antiviral cytokines such as interferon-gamma and more of a distinct set of Interleukins (notably IL-4, IL-5, and IL-13), which are able to stimulate quite different cell types and functions. Clearly these did not evolve simply to promote allergy—the driving force appears to be host defence against worms. Worm infection is more complex than bacterial, fungal, or viral, since the invading pathogen is multi-cellular and is orders of magnitude larger in size than the immune cells fighting it, and thus is not readily phagocytosed. Although in modern Western societies, encounters with worm infections are rare, in earlier stages of human evolution, worm infection would have represented an enormous burden—and it remains so in some parts of the world. Thus, a robust defence against worms is essential and requires a combination of effectors mobilized through the Type 2 response.

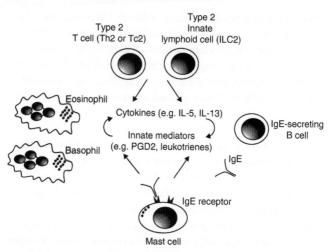

22. The diagram indicates some of the important cells and mediators involved in Type 2 responses. The triggering antigens which are recognized by Type 2 T cells and specific IgE include harmless proteins (e.g. from house dust mites) as well as drugs and insect venoms.

One key set of cells which are induced as part of this process are *eosinophils*. These are bone marrow derived and related to neutrophils, but possess a different content of granules and thus are readily distinguished. These granules contain specific, highly potent molecules which can digest and attack tissues, including worms—these include reactive oxygen species, protease enzymes, and pore-forming proteins that attack cell membranes. They also secrete a large set of mediators which recruit further cells to the site and activate them. Excess levels of eosinophils in the blood is one hallmark of worm infection—it is also a hallmark of allergy.

Another important mediator of allergy driven by the Type 2 response is the development of a particular type of antibody called the E class—*IgE*. Like high levels of eosinophils, high levels of IgE are associated strongly with allergy. IgE is no different from any other antibody at the antigen recognition end. However, the molecule is distinct in that it can activate a set of receptors present on specific subsets of immune cells called *mast cells*. If a mast cell with activated receptors encounters an antigen—for example, in the skin or airways—there is a rapid activation of the cell itself, resulting in a burst of inflammatory signals. Mast cell activation is highly potent as the cell contains pre-formed molecules, such as histamines, which leads to immediate inflammatory responses in the tissue—this is manifest as local swelling and irritation. Massive mast cell release can lead to very profound general effects—so-called *anaphylaxis*, where there may be a sudden drop in blood pressure, generalized swelling particularly of sensitive areas such as the face and tongue, and a rash. This response can be brought on by exposure to any antigen to which IgE has developed at sufficient levels, including proteins in insect stings, drugs, and food.

Allergic responses are commonly seen as organ-specific diseases, such as hay fever, asthma, or eczema. Often these are linked together within an individual or within families, and indeed there is a strong genetic predisposition to such diseases. Although many of the genes involved relate to the immune response, not all of them do. For eczema, mutations in the filaggrin gene lead to a subtle disruption of the skin barrier—exactly how this leads to allergy is not known, but it is likely that it allows exposure to more antigens or a change in the context in which the immune system encounters an antigen, thus raising its awareness and promoting a Type 2 response.

Other mutations affect molecules involved specifically in the activation of different cell subsets involved in the Type 2 reaction, for example CRTH2. CRTH2 is a surface receptor for prostaglandin D2—one of the important lipid mediators released by mast cells. CRTH2 is found on Type 2 T cells, on eosinophils, on basophils (which are closely related), and also on innate lymphoid cells which have a Type 2 bias. It is thus a distinct marker of the Type 2 subset and furthermore a target for drugs which can block prostaglandin signalling. Prostaglandins and their lipid relatives, leukotrienes, are involved in a range of inflammatory processes, and blockade of the action of leukotrienes by the drug Montelukast has long been used as a treatment for asthma.

Although a wide range of cells are involved in allergic responses, they share a few key pathways, and signalling molecules (such as Prostaglandin D2 or Interleukin 5), which are rather distinct from those encountered in other immune settings. This offers some hope that we can find treatments for asthma that are more targeted. Allergic asthma results from ongoing Type 2 responses in the lung, which lead to inflammation of the airways and constriction of the airways. These are related but distinct features. Currently treatment relies in most cases on the use of inhaled steroids to suppress local inflammation and compounds related to adrenaline to improve the airway constriction. However, if the disease is severe, steroids must be given at high doses orally or intravenously to keep the airways open, and this is associated with long-term side effects (bone thinning, immune suppression, weight gain).

Approaches to specifically turn off Type 2 responses which underpin this severe disease are still needed, although biologic agents which block, for example, Interleukin 5 represent one interesting approach. It is also possible in some cases of allergy to reprogramme the immune response and replace the Type 2 response with a less dangerous one. This can be done by a process of *desensitization* whereby a tiny dose of the antigen is given in the skin, and this dosing is repeated and built up over a long period of time. What is observed is that IgE levels (e.g. from bee venom) to the antigen drop, while IgG4 responses may replace these. IgG4 is an interesting molecule which has little activatory function and may serve as a blocking or inhibitory antibody. This therapy has in fact been in place for over a century, developed well before a clear understanding of the immune mechanisms was in place—but the same is true for vaccines.

There is still much to learn about allergy—for instance the reason why an individual develops a particular allergic response to a given antigen is not well understood. Like auto-immunity there will be a component from the genetic polymorphisms the person has inherited and the environment to which they are exposed, including their microbiome. One prevalent theory which suggests a specific role for environmental exposure is the *hygiene hypothesis*, whereby exposure to a high microbial burden in childhood reduces the chance of developing an allergy. This is somewhat controversial but has been put forward to explain the rise in allergic diseases in Western societies.

Certainly there are data which support the idea that the greater the diversity of pathogens to which children are exposed (e.g. living on a farm increases this substantially), the lower the risk of allergy. In a study of the Amish and Hutterite communities in the USA, it was found that although the two groups were very closely matched in many ways, the Amish children had a much lower incidence of asthma. It turns out that the Amish communities used traditional farming practices as opposed to the modern industrialized techniques adopted by the Hutterites, and the environment in Amish homes was characterized by a much greater range and burden of microbes. How exactly this microbial exposure may work, by diverting or training the immune response, is not fully understood, but it is another example of how the microbiome may have a pervasive influence on immune development.

Chapter 7

The immune system v2.0: biological and immune therapies

In the previous chapters we have discussed the basic building blocks of the immune system, how they work as a team, and what happens when the teamwork breaks down. This basic knowledge can be applied, however, to influence outcomes of disease—both immunological and beyond. In this chapter we will discuss three major inter-related areas where our knowledge of immunology is being applied to current challenges: boosting immunity in the case of vaccines, harnessing immunity for cancer treatment, and the development of novel treatments for blocking immunity and auto-immunity. We will also look at the issues linked to the ageing immune response and how these may be corrected to treat or prevent disease.

Boosting immunity and vaccines

First let's consider how to boost immune responses, and perhaps the most obvious application is in the field of vaccines. Vaccines have had an enormous impact on human health for centuries, and the immunological principles which underlie them are increasingly well understood—but we still lack effective vaccines for major infections such as HIV, TB, and malaria. Why is this and what can be done? What these three infections have in common, and is also common to other complex vaccine targets such as HCV and CMV, is their capacity to persist. Infections such as influenza,

Haemophilus influenzae, and measles tend not to set up a persistent infection in an otherwise healthy host and the immunity induced is robust—so a vaccine approach which generates high levels of antibody against the prevailing strains can provide *protective immunity*. For influenza the challenge is to establish which strains pose the threat, and there is a wide range with some avian strains being very dangerous indeed if they cross into human hosts, but the issue is nevertheless the same. For the current influenza vaccines, providing the proteins derived from the relevant virus type circulating that season (using virus grown on chicken eggs), together with an adjuvant, which enhances the innate immune response, is usually sufficient to induce protective levels of neutralizing antibody. For measles, which is an attenuated version of the natural virus, this immunity is lifelong.

However, as we have seen for HIV, generation of antibodies against the viral envelope can neutralize some strains but is readily escaped by others and provides only limited protection. One trial (RV144, in Thailand) which was designed to induce antibodies against the HIV envelope has shown partial success in preventing infection and has raised hopes that effective antibodies can be raised, but there is a long way to go before this can be used, as the level of protection was only 30 per cent. Further attempts to optimize the antigen used, and to focus the antibody response on regions which can neutralize multiple variants, may enhance this.

Alternative approaches are hoped to harness the T cell response in providing protection. This would be relying on the CD8+ T cells to clear infection from already infected cells and so is quite a different approach from that used in the vaccines mentioned earlier. Such approaches have been tried, but unsuccessfully, and there were concerns raised that the vaccines may even increase the chances of infection in people with HIV. It may be that the T cells need to be targeted to the right peptides in the virus.

One approach from the lab of Louis Picker has been to use CMV as a *vector* (carrier virus) to deliver the HIV proteins. The CMV used in these experiments can disable some aspects of MHC Class I presentation, which apparently forces the immune system to use alternative presenting molecules, in this case a molecule in humans known as HLA-E.

HLA-E is not polymorphic and presents a limited set of peptides, normally to NK cells—but in the context of this vaccine, which to date has only been used in monkeys, it can present viral peptides. The immune responses to these peptides are very strong and quite distinct from the normal immune response, and they can be remarkably effective in suppressing infection. These experiments provide some proof-of-principle that T cell-based approaches could work, if this can be translated safely into human studies.

Virally vectored vaccines—that is, vaccines where the target pathogen is presented to the immune system using another virus (see Figure 23)—do have huge potential. It is possible to engineer safe viruses which can present the target antigens (from e.g. TB, Zika virus, or Ebola) to the immune system, and some of these (e.g. adenoviruses) are able to prime extremely vigorous immune responses. This means it is not necessary to grow the pathogens in the lab, and the immune response can in theory be targeted specifically to the regions of interest. It is also possible to use DNA itself as a vaccine—the injected DNA will be used by the cell to generate the protein of interest and there may be a sufficient innate response to the vaccine to prime new T and B cells. DNA vaccines work very effectively in mice but relatively poorly in humans—indeed one of the handicaps of this area is that many vaccine approaches that work well in the laboratory fail to induce strong immune responses in human volunteers.

So, some of the difficulties in generating vaccines against complex pathogens arise from failure to understand what type of immunity is protective and what target to hit, and some arise from failing to

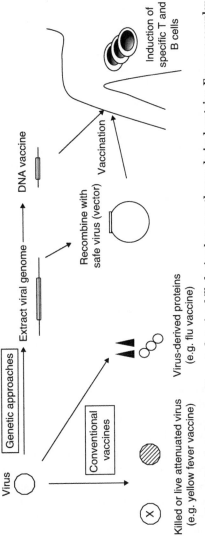

23. Conventional vaccines use attenuated strains, killed microbes, or pathogen-derived proteins. For more complex or dangerous pathogens a genetic approach may provide an alternative vaccine strategy.

be able to induce immune responses using current approaches. Of the two, the latter is easier to address since better understanding of innate responses and antigen presentation coupled with an increasingly diverse array of molecular tools to deliver antigens could solve this issue. Defining protective immunity and trying to reproduce it exactly is much harder—even using animal models which represent human disease—and so it may still be a matter of trial and error in some cases. Two particularly complex diseases which currently lack effective vaccine strategies are malaria and TB. These share some features with HIV: malaria has very high levels of variability, which make it very hard for the host's responses to keep up with the pathogen, while TB sets up a reservoir of latent infection antigens which is very hard to eliminate and represents a continuous threat of potential reinfection.

Immunity to malaria is actually possible to develop through continuous exposure over time—infection of children and infants is very dangerous and associated with severe illness, but adults from communities in areas where malaria is endemic, such as in sub-Saharan Africa, may suffer minimal or no clinical impact from a malarial infection. Much effort has been expended in defining the mechanisms that limit the infection in such individuals (interestingly such effective immunity is lost if the individuals move away from an endemic area) and a vaccine—RTS,S—has been generated as a result. This vaccine, which uses HBV to present malarial antigens to the immune system is, however, only partially effective in infants and the effect wears off over time, so there is certainly more work to be done here. Malaria parasites have a complex lifestyle which includes a key stage passing through the liver after the mosquito bite, before emerging and passing into red blood cells. Where the infection in the liver can be blocked this provides very effective immunity. Approaches to direct anti-malaria T cell responses into the liver using virally vectored vaccines or even whole, irradiated malaria parasites can provide quite efficient immunity (see Figure 24).

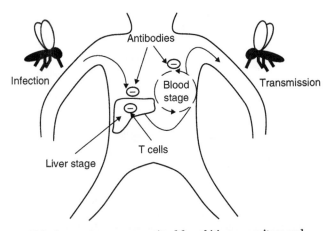

24. Malaria parasites are transmitted from biting mosquitoes and must enter the liver in order to establish infection. Antibodies and T cells induced by vaccines and natural exposure can block this process at different points.

TB is caused by Mtb (see Chapter 2) and spread largely by aerosol droplets from infected individuals presenting with a productive cough. The organism is present in about a third of the world's population, and the key step in its life cycle is its ability to set up long-term latency in macrophages, the major cell it infects. The bacterium is able to manipulate the intracellular environment of the macrophage to enhance its survival and evade immune elimination. Since it is intracellular, the key immune responses are delivered by T cells, and deficits in T cell immunity can lead to reactivation of TB. T cells secrete cytokines such as interferon-gamma and TNF-alpha which activate the macrophages and enhance the elimination. This cross-talk between T cells and macrophages leads to the development of a *granuloma*—a complex mass of immune cells at the centre of which is embedded the bacterium driving the response (see Figure 25).

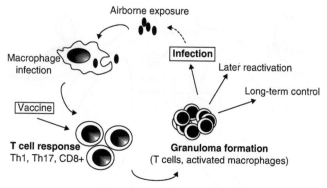

25. *Mycobacterium tuberculosis* (Mtb) **is taken up by macrophages. In most cases Mtb persists in a granuloma and it can reactivate at a later date. If T cell immunity is poor, further spread of Mtb within the lung can occur.**

A T cell vaccine against TB has existed for nearly a century in the form of BCG developed at the Pasteur Institute in Paris. This vaccine—which is based on an attenuated strain of TB developed in culture—does indeed generate high levels of T cell response against Mtb antigens. It has also been shown to be highly effective in preventing disease in infants, where it can be very severe, spreading throughout the body including to the brain (i.e. meningitis). However, BCG is much less obviously effective in adults and no new vaccine has been developed since. The reasons for this are not yet clear, but one issue is that we do not yet know what the key mediators of protection are and therefore what the vaccine should target. Once we have a clear target the methods to induce T cell immunity in humans are now well advanced and so new TB vaccine strategies could provide a breakthrough prevention of this major, global health problem.

It is clearly important to develop new vaccines. One high priority is RSV (see also Chapter 4) which is a widespread, indeed ubiquitous, virus to which we are all exposed and which causes severe disease in young infants. A vaccine against RSV would be of enormous benefit around the world, but an attempt to make one in the 1960s was associated with increased disease and also death in those vaccinated. It is likely that this resulted from an aberrant Type 2 immune response generated against the vaccine, which was developed from a live virus that had been rendered inactive by a chemical, formalin. Thus an enhanced immune response was not protective but rather led to hypersensitivity to the virus and increased lung inflammation.

Further attempts to make vaccines against RSV are nevertheless underway, using our increased knowledge of the immune system to avoid this dangerous problem either by using viral vectors to deliver the RSV antigens, or by vaccinating the mother, allowing her to pass on her boosted IgG antibodies to the infant and thus passively protect them. The infant's levels of protective antibody will drop over time but this means infection at the most vulnerable age can be avoided. There is emerging evidence that RSV also causes disease in the elderly, when immune responses wane (discussed later in this chapter), and here vaccines to boost antibodies and T cells against RSV could prevent serious infection in this age group.

Overall the development of vaccines against common diseases has saved countless lives and will continue to do so—they not only protect the individual vaccinated but beyond that provide *herd immunity*, limiting the spread of serious infections. This issue of herd immunity has come to the fore in recent controversies over the use of specific vaccines. Because vaccines are given to healthy individuals, the benefits of protection have to be weighed against the risks of possible adverse effects. Fortunately, because the impact of some of these infections is very great, and the risk from the vaccines is small, this equation comes down well in favour of benefit. If the same balance and outcome can be achieved using the next generation of vaccines against major pathogens such as those mentioned in this chapter, this has the potential to impact positively on millions of lives.

Harnessing immunity and cancer immunotherapy

Boosting immunity is not only of relevance to infections but also to cancer (Figure 26). One of the most exciting breakthroughs in the last decade has been the development of new techniques to harness anti-cancer immune responses for patient benefit. The evidence from HIV (and other immunosuppressive states) already suggested that the immune response plays a major role in controlling cancers, primarily those that are driven by viruses. However, most cancers do not contain viral proteins as potential targets but are simply mutated versions of self. Given the layers of tolerance described in the last chapter, immune responses to self are highly attenuated—additionally cancers behave somewhat like infections, undergoing selection to avoid elimination.

Thus developing an effective cellular immune response against cancers could be considered a very difficult proposition. On the

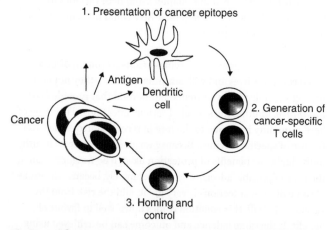

26. Several features of cancers serve to limit cancer-specific immunity. These negative effects work both on the induction of the immune response (dendritic cell) and also at the effector stage (in the tumour micro-environment).

other hand there have been intermittent successes in this field, where some patients have demonstrated a striking response to vaccination or the transfer of specific T cells, which has led to continued optimism regarding this approach. In looking at outcomes from cancer, and studying the cells and genes in the tumours themselves, there are signs that the greater the immune response in the tumour, the better the survival of the patient. Recent data used to examine outcomes from thousands of patients with thirty different types of cancer revealed that the single gene in the tumours most closely linked to a good outcome was an immune gene—KLRB1—encoding for CD161, a molecule expressed on subsets of T cells and NK cells with enhanced functions.

What might such T cells be recognizing within a cancer? One answer lies in analysing the cancer itself, which is a result of genetic mutations in the DNA of the host cells. Each time a significant mutation is made, a new peptide target is created that was not present in the thymus and where tolerance has not been previously induced. If such a peptide can be bound to the patient's MHC molecule and presented to the T cell, then it can represent a *neo-epitope*—a suitable target for recognition and killing of the tumour cell. Interestingly, some tumours where this process of mutation is accelerated (due to loss of proofreading of the cell's replication machinery) are actually better controlled, and associated with a more vigorous immune response—likely targeting the large set of neo-epitopes generated. With new methods of sequencing of cancer genomes now available, it is possible to identify the neo-epitopes which are present in an individual patient's cancer. In principle targeting these with a vaccine approach could lead to bespoke cancer therapies.

However, the T cell responses also need to overcome the tolerance effects present in tissues and in particular the checkpoints provided by inhibitory molecules. This is the area where the recent ability to block such checkpoints with monoclonal antibodies has had the biggest impact. Blockade of inhibitory molecules such as PD1 and CTLA4 can have a huge impact on cancer control—in combination (and without other treatment) these can lead to marked extension of disease-free survival in patients with advanced melanoma, one of the most aggressive forms of cancer. Melanomas are an interesting tumour as they possess well-established targets for the immune system and have been known to respond to immune therapies in the past. Checkpoint blockade is now being applied to a range of other tumour types, such as lung cancer and renal cancers. The downside, as may be expected, is the induction of auto-immune phenomena (gut inflammation is particularly common), but given the prognosis from the cancer itself, these can be largely accepted if appropriately controlled.

There are a number of mechanisms which regulate T cell functions in healthy tissues and tumours, so it is hoped that this success can be built upon to provide a range of options to liberate anti-tumour responses in future—but this approach does depend on the presence of a potentially active T cell response. Thus it may also be coupled with efforts to boost the anti-tumour response through vaccines (as described in this chapter) or using infusions of lymphocytes—so-called cellular therapies.

One novel approach to cellular therapy is the creation of so-called chimeric antigen receptor (CAR-T) cells, where the TCR has been engineered to respond specifically to the patient's cancer. This can target new T cells to the cancer where they are activated and display effector functions. This targeting can be made exquisitely specific by engineering an antibody domain onto the TCR—thus this does not rely on peptide presentation of a processed peptide, but rather expression of a cancer antigen on the cell surface. Antibody binding to such targets is very specific and very strong. This approach is also interesting as the T cells may remain circulating and provide long-term protection against recurrence. Similar approaches are being attempted using engineered soluble

TCRs which have been selected for their ability to very strongly bind to a tumour target (normally TCRs are relatively weak, since strong binders are eliminated in the thymus). These can be designed so that when engaged with their target they can recruit effector T cells and activate them directly at the site of the tumour, thus hugely increasing the numbers of cells involved in the anti-tumour response.

Blocking immunity and biological therapies

On the one hand, our understanding of the mechanisms of tolerance can allow us to break them and enhance inflammation in the case of cancer responses. On the other, our knowledge of the basic mechanisms of inflammation can suggest strategies to block auto-immune responses. The most interesting new approach to such a blockade relies on adapting the immune response itself to generate *biological therapies* based on monoclonal antibodies, developed by César Milstein and Georges Köhler, who shared the Nobel Prize for this work with Niels Jerne.

Monoclonal antibodies are derived from the normal antibody response, which contains many different forms of antibody response even to the same antigen. To make a single, purified form, Köhler and Milstein fused B cells with *immortalized* cancer cells (i.e. cells which can keep on dividing and therefore growing indefinitely in the lab) to create a series of *hybridomas*. These immortalized cells all secrete an antibody, but each cell makes an antibody of a distinct and unique design. By doing this at scale, and then screening the resultant hybridomas for binding to the antigen of choice (in the original study it was sheep red blood cells, but it can be anything which evokes an antibody response), it is possible to select those hybridomas with the correct specificity. Since hybridomas are immortalized this allows immunologists to make almost unlimited quantities of highly purified and specific antibodies to targets of their choice. This technology is still used, although newer, more flexible alternatives have been developed.

Monoclonal antibodies allow for precise blockading of specific aspects of the immune system or targeting of pathogens. Although these tools were developed by Milstein and Köhler in the 1970s, it took some time for their therapeutic potential to be realized. The leader of this pack was the development of monoclonal antibodies to Tumor Necrosis Factor alpha (TNFa). This molecule is highly pro-inflammatory and is involved in many and diverse auto-immune and inflammatory responses as well as being critical in host defence. Monoclonal therapy for TNFa was tested initially in the context of sepsis—a severe condition of bloodstream infections associated with a very high mortality rate. Like many therapies for this condition, it was not successful. However, Marc Feldman and Ravinder Maini, who had been working on TNFa in RA and had shown the effects of blockade in the test tube, were able to repurpose this treatment—known as *Infliximab*—in a small trial of patients with this disabling condition. The results from this trial in 1992 were remarkably effective, with a substantial proportion of patients benefiting from the monoclonal antibody, and paving the way for a flood of such biological treatments in the following decades. TNFa blockade (using Infliximab and other biological approaches) is now used in treating a wide range of inflammatory conditions, including IBD (Crohn's disease and ulcerative colitis), ankylosing spondylitis, and psoriatic arthritis.

Biological therapies allow the pinpoint blockade of specific pathways involved in inflammation, thus avoiding the use of very broad immunosuppressive therapies such as steroids. However, there are side effects which may be predicted from the role of these molecules in host defence. TNFa is critically important in the control of TB, and even though other immune defence mechanisms remain intact, those treated with this agent are at risk of reactivating this infection. Also, although the molecule has been engineered to be 'humanized' (it was originally developed in a mouse), it can still, in some patients, attract an antibody response which limits its effectiveness. Not all patients with RA (or the other diseases mentioned) respond to such drugs. This suggests that although RA appears to be one disease, there may be different underlying mechanisms at work in different patients—so further stratification of patients for these expensive and potentially dangerous therapies is needed—a common theme in modern medicine.

Beyond TNFa, a number of other cytokine pathways can be targeted by monoclonal antibodies. The Type 17 pathway has been mentioned previously as a contributor to inflammatory disease, as well as protecting against infection by bacteria and yeasts. Blockade of IL-23, a cytokine that promotes such responses, is also effective in inflammatory diseases of the joints and bowel. Interestingly blockade of IL-17 itself is effective in treating ankylosing spondylitis, an inflammatory disease of the spine, and also in psoriasis—diseases which share a number of genetic risk factors with each other and with IBD. However, IL-17 blockade in IBD actually made the inflammation worse, possibly by reducing the host response to bacteria and thus accentuating the original injury. In some ways, therefore, these clinical studies are experiments themselves, revealing further aspects of the underlying disease once one pathway has been blocked; or revealing the role of a specific pathway in host defence.

The ability to target and specifically block an inflammatory pathway in patients with chronic inflammation has been hugely attractive to scientists and companies, and the list of products now in trial or available for use is very long. Monoclonal antibodies to block other inflammatory cytokines or their receptors such as for Interleukins 1b and 6 can also be used to treat arthritis and may represent alternatives for those who do not respond to TNFa blockade. Blockade of IL-5 and potentially IL-13 represent interventions for allergy and asthma. There is plenty of potential to influence these inflammatory conditions, although the development of such agents is very costly and so care must be taken in choosing the right targets.

Other approaches based on monoclonal therapy include cell depletion—indeed Campath 1, targeting T cells through their surface receptor CD52, was one of the first such treatments developed by Herman Waldmann in Cambridge. Now known as Alemtuzumab, this depleting antibody can have a substantial impact on the course of MS and is one of the few therapies which is really effective in this disease. Depletion of cells using monoclonals can also be effective in cancer. Alemtuzumab can be used for specific lymphatic tumours, to destroy the proliferating lymphocytes, but more importantly targeting of the CD20 molecule by the antibody Rituximab on B cells is a powerful treatment for a range of lymphomas. Rituximab, by depleting B cells (most of which express the CD20 molecule and are targets for the drug), can also reset the immune system and can be used to turn off antibody responses in RA and a range of auto-immune conditions. The story for these molecules, like that of Infliximab mentioned earlier, is informative—although introduced for a single condition or application, they can be turned to a variety of uses, including in relatively rare or 'orphan' conditions where specific drugs are unlikely to be developed.

Monoclonal antibodies and biological therapies can also be used to block the migration of cells to specific tissues. Vedolizumab is a blocker of specific *integrins* used to allow cells to home in on the gut where it is active in the treatment of IBD. Natulizumab is a related molecule but it impacts on the homing action of lymphocytes to both gut and brain, and can be used to treat MS. Failure to allow lymphocytes to survey the brain tissue, however, does not come without risk, since rare cases of a severe viral infection caused by JC virus can occur. This is also seen in advanced HIV patients, linked to profound immunosuppression and with a very poor outcome. Such viral reactivations do occur in other settings, and while some are predictable and preventable (such as reactivation of chronic HBV), many are not, and care must be taken even with such targeted therapies (see Figure 27).

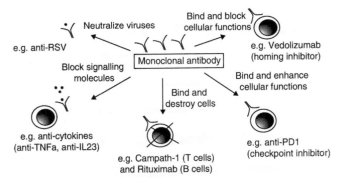

27. Monoclonal antibodies allow for precise blockade of specific aspects of the immune system or targeting of pathogens. The ability to bind and kill cells can be used for immunotherapy and cancer therapy.

Turning off immune responses is not only required for inflammatory diseases but also for transplantation, and here monoclonal antibodies also play a role. Additionally, attempts have been made to induce tolerance using a range of techniques. One interesting idea based on cell therapy is to transfer in regulatory T cells. CD4+ T cells which express high levels of the IL-2 receptor CD25, marking out Tregs, can be sorted from peripheral blood, cultured in the laboratory, and transfused into the recipient. These cells may also be treated in vitro to enhance their ability to suppress. In pre-clinical studies this approach has been highly effective and there is much enthusiasm to translate it into human use, even though there will be many practical barriers to overcome. Treg therapy may also have a role in auto-immune diseases and potentially has the advantage of providing a relatively specific attenuation of the aberrant immune response without the risk of severe infection.

Inflammation and ageing ('inflammageing')

Finally, looking to the future, one issue we currently face is that of diseases of ageing, and in these the immune response may need

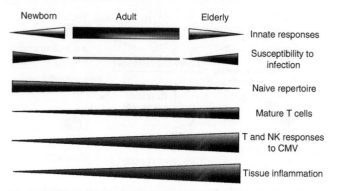

Newborn	Adult	Elderly	
			Innate responses
			Susceptibility to infection
			Naive repertoire
			Mature T cells
			T and NK responses to CMV
			Tissue inflammation

28. Ageing is associated with many immunological changes which affect susceptibility to infection and regulation of inflammation. CMV infection drives very strong immune responses and has been associated with some of these effects.

tuning either up or down (see Figure 28). Alzheimer's disease is not considered an auto-immune disease like RA or MS, but there is increasing evidence, from studies of those affected and genetic analysis of large populations, that the immune response is involved. TREM2 is one such gene which is implicated in Alzheimer's disease and appears to influence the function of microglial cells—related to macrophages—in the brain. Exactly how TREM2 influences the development or progression of the dementia process is not currently understood, but it provides a potential new therapeutic opportunity to intervene in this devastating and prevalent illness.

Ageing itself may be accelerated by inflammation—so-called 'inflammageing'. This is a very complicated area because a number of factors are involved and distinguishing healthy ageing from premature senescence is not simple. One factor which may play a role is chronic inflammation due to infection. A culprit in many studies is CMV, a virus carried by most of the world's population and one where its capacity to lie dormant and then reactivate means that continuous immune surveillance is required. This in itself leads to a marked skewing of immune responses due to the number of lymphocytes recruited to this effort, and has been linked to premature senescence of the immune system, with loss of responsiveness. There is accruing data that loss of control over CMV, in a subset of individuals, leads to viral reactivation and inflammation. Since the virus is able to survive in the linings of blood vessels (endothelial cells), this could contribute to vascular disease. Further studies with large populations to address this specific hypothesis are needed—if this is indeed found to be true, then it may provide an interesting opportunity to interrupt the process of ageing.

Furthermore, developing vaccine strategies and other interventions to maintain an effective immune response in an ageing population will be of increasing importance in future. One recently explored idea is to focus on the metabolism of immune cells, specifically a process known as *autophagy*, or self-eating. Autophagy is a mechanism for recycling cell contents in order to maintain cell survival and is triggered by starvation. Much data have accrued to show that stimulating autophagy can improve lifespan. In the case of lymphocytes, autophagy is required to maintain long-lived memory—in one experiment, triggering autophagy in aged mice, which had markedly impaired T cell memory, using a molecule called spermidine, led to a marked improvement in memory T cell responses. This suggests that immune ageing processes are at least partially reversible and that simple interventions (spermidine, for example, is found in food) could assist this rejuvenation process. Autophagy can also be induced by many other means, including calorie restriction and exercise. So there may be multiple ways to influence this critical pathway and boost the ageing immune system. There are likely other pathways involved that limit immunity or immune regulation with age, but which are currently poorly explored.

Interestingly, autophagy is highly regulated by diet and exercise. The overall impact of nutritional status on such basic cellular processes is likely very important and the role of metabolic regulation of the immune system is of great significance. For example, micronutrients such as vitamins and minerals may modulate effector vs regulatory functions of T cells. Diabetes, which is an increasing problem in Western ageing populations, is linked with depression of immune function and increased susceptibility to infection. Further mechanistic and clinical studies are needed to better define whether specific interventions in diet and lifestyle can impact on immune responses and inflammatory processes in populations of all ages.

The future of the immune system

In this book we have examined the basic building blocks of the immune response, as we have inherited them through evolution, and how they coordinate their functions to balance aggression (against dangerous pathogens) with tolerance (of self and the microbiome). The job is normally done so well that we ignore its daily impact on our lives—only noticing it when it is impaired. In the first chapter, we discussed how the immune system involves the whole body and how we are increasingly aware that inflammatory processes are involved in many diseases, from heart disease through to cancer and dementia.

Evolution likely tuned our immune system to get us through only the first few decades of life so that the issues discussed earlier in this chapter may be a consequence of this early-age bias. The diseases we face globally still include many infectious challenges—such as HIV, malaria, and TB. Prevention and cure of these diseases will rely on better understanding of the targets of the immune system and on developing more practical systems for the induction of protective T and B cell immunity. This is an extension of the work that has been going on since Jenner and then Pasteur, the pioneers of vaccination, with increasing levels of refinement, driven by better understanding of basic immunology and microbiology. Here, harnessing the immune system through vaccine development has been enormously successful.

The diseases of the 21st century, particularly in the developed world, are dominated by cardiovascular disease and cancer, with dementia and diseases of old age emerging as population structures change. This is a different challenge for immunologists, but since the immune system involves the whole body and many important pathologies it is a challenge that must be met. The ability to specifically block inflammatory pathways—using small-molecule drugs or biological molecules based on monoclonal antibody technology—provides us with an important set of tools to modulate immune responses in these new settings. Given the enormous advances these approaches have made in classical auto-immune and inflammatory diseases such as RA and IBD, the new set of challenges can be approached with some optimism. Tuning or retraining the immune system to operate effectively in old age—that is, boosting immunity against infection while preventing chronic inflammation—is too complex a task for those in this field to tackle alone, and will need input from those in many other fields. However, as we dissect the immunological pathways involved in such diseases this will continue to provide new opportunities for treatment and ultimately prevention of these and other such conditions facing all of us as individuals and as a society.

Further reading

Books

Daniel M. Davis (2014) *The Compatibility Gene* (Penguin).

Arthur M. Silverstein (2009) *A History of Immunology*, 2nd edition (Academic Press).

Kenneth Murphy (2014) *Janeway's Immunobiology*, 8th edition (Garland Science).

Raif Geha and Luigi Notarangelo (2016) *Case Studies in Immunology—A Clinical Companion*, 7th edition (Garland Science).

Lauren Sompayrac (2012) *How the Immune System Works*, 4th edition (Blackwell Science).

Abul Abbas, Andrew H. Lichtman, and Shiv Pillai (2014) *Cellular and Molecular Immunology*, 8th edition (Saunders).

Peter Parham (2014) *The Immune System*, 4th edition (Garland Science).

Gordon MacPherson and Jon Austyn (2012) *Exploring Immunology—Concepts and Evidence*, 1st edition (Wiley VCH).

Warren E. Levinson (2014) *Review of Medical Microbiology and Immunology*, 13th edition (McGraw-Hill).

David Male, Jonathan Brostoff, David Roth, and Ivan Roitt (eds) (2012) *Immunology*, 8th edition (Saunders).

William Paul (2012) *Fundamental Immunology*, 7th edition (Lippincott Williams and Wilkins).

David Warrell, Tim Cox, and John Firth (eds) (2010) *Oxford Textbook of Medicine*, 5th edition (Oxford University Press). (Chapter 5, 'Immune Mechanisms', ed. Graham Ogg.)

Reviews

The field of immunology moves fast. The following journals publish up-to-date review articles on the subjects covered in this book, listed on PubMed (<https://www.ncbi.nlm.nih.gov/pubmed>):

Advances in Immunology <http://www.sciencedirect.com/science/bookseries/00652776>.

Annual Review of Immunology <http://www.annualreviews.org/journal/immunol>.

Current Opinion in Immunology <https://www.journals.elsevier.com/current-opinion-in-immunology>.

Immunological Reviews <http://onlinelibrary.wiley.com/journal/10.1111/(ISSN)1600-065X>.

Nature Reviews Immunology <http://www.nature.com/nri/index.html>.

Nature Reviews Microbiology <http://www.nature.com/nrmicro/index.html>.

Trends in Immunology <https://www.journals.elsevier.com/trends-in-immunology/>.

See also

R. M. Zinkernagel (1996) 'Immunology Taught by Viruses', *Science* 271: 173–8.

R. E. Phillips (2002) 'Immunology Taught by Darwin', *Nature Immunology* 3: 987–9.

M. M. Davis (2012) 'Immunology Taught by Humans', *Science Translational Medicine* 4: 117fs2. doi: 10.1126/scitranslmed.3003385.

J. L. Casanova, L. Abel, and L. Quintana-Murci (2013) 'Immunology Taught by Human Genetics', *Cold Spring Harbor Symposia on Quantitative Biology* 78: 157–72. doi: 10.1101/sqb.2013.78.019968.

Index

Index

119

SOCIAL MEDIA
Very Short Introduction

Join our community
www.oup.com/vsi

- Join us online at the official Very Short Introductions **Facebook** page.
- Access the thoughts and musings of our authors with our online **blog**.
- Sign up for our monthly **e-newsletter** to receive information on all new titles publishing that month.
- Browse the full range of Very Short Introductions online.
- Read **extracts** from the Introductions for free.
- If you are a teacher or lecturer you can order inspection copies quickly and simply via our website.

CANCER
A Very Short Introduction
Nick James

Cancer research is a major economic activity. There are constant improvements in treatment techniques that result in better cure rates and increased quality and quantity of life for those with the disease, yet stories of breakthroughs in a cure for cancer are often in the media. In this *Very Short Introduction* Nick James, founder of the CancerHelp UK website, examines the trends in diagnosis and treatment of the disease, as well as its economic consequences. Asking what cancer is and what causes it, he considers issues surrounding expensive drug development, what can be done to reduce the risk of developing cancer, and the use of complementary and alternative therapies.

HIV/AIDS
A Very Short Introduction
Alan Whiteside

HIV/AIDS is without doubt the worst epidemic to hit humankind since the Black Death. The first case was identified in 1981; by 2004 it was estimated that about 40 million people were living with the disease, and about 20 million had died. The news is not all bleak though. There have been unprecedented breakthroughs in understanding diseases and developing drugs. Because the disease is so closely linked to sexual activity and drug use, the need to understand and change behaviour has caused us to reassess what it means to be human and how we should operate in the globalising world. This *Very Short Introduction* provides an introduction to the disease, tackling the science, the international and local politics, the fascinating demographics, and the devastating consequences of the disease, and explores how we have — and must — respond.

'It won't make you an expert. But you'll know what you're talking about and you'll have a better idea of all the work we still have to do to wrestle this monster to the ground.'

Aids-free world website.

EPIDEMIOLOGY
A Very Short Introduction
Rodolfo Saracci

Epidemiology has had an impact on many areas of medicine;
and lung cancer, to the origin and spread of new epidemics.
and lung cancer, to the origin and spread of new epidemics.
However, it is often poorly understood, largely due to
misrepresentations in the media. In this *Very Short Introduction*
Rodolfo Saracci dispels some of the myths surrounding the
study of epidemiology. He provides a general explanation of
the principles behind clinical trials, and explains the nature of
basic statistics concerning disease. He also looks at the ethical
and political issues related to obtaining and using information
concerning patients, and trials involving placebos.

AUTISM
A Very Short Introduction
Uta Frith

This *Very Short Introduction* offers a clear statement on what is currently known about autism and Asperger syndrome. Explaining the vast array of different conditions that hide behind these two labels, and looking at symptoms from the full spectrum of autistic disorders, it explores the possible causes for the apparent rise in autism and also evaluates the links with neuroscience, psychology, brain development, genetics, and environmental causes including MMR and Thimerosal. This short, authoritative, and accessible book also explores the psychology behind social impairment and savantism and sheds light on what it is like to live inside the mind of the sufferer.

www.oup.com/vsi